Fortify Your Immune System Naturally

Dr. Kari Koester-Loesche

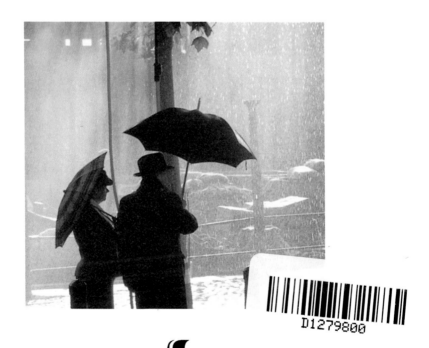

D1279800

Sterling Publishing Co., Inc.   New York

Translated from German by John S. Lewis and Ruth A. Lewis. This book has been carefully produced; however, neither the author, the translator, nor the publisher is responsible for the use of the information given in the book. Anyone with a medical problem should consult a physician. Portions of this book have been revised for the English edition.

Library of Congress Cataloging-in-Publication Data

Köster-Lösche, Kari, 1946–
    [Immunsystem näturlich stärken.   English]
    Fortify your immune system naturally / Kari Köster-Lösche.
      p. cm.
    "Originally published in Germany under the title: Das Immunsystem näturlich stärken"–T.p. verso.
    Includes index.
    ISBN 0-8069-4215-0
    1. Health.   2. Immunity.   3. Immune system.   4. Nutrition.
I. Title.
RA776.K696913   1998
616.07'9–dc21   98-3370
                                            CIP

10 9 8 7 6 5 4 3 2 1

Published by Sterling Publishing Company, Inc.
387 Park Avenue South, New York, N.Y. 10016
Originally published in Germany under the title *Das Immunsystem natürlich stärken* by Dr. Kari Köster-Lösche
©1995 by Südwest Verlag GmbH & Co. KG, Munich, Germany
English translation ©1998 by Sterling Publishing Co.
Distributed in Canada by Sterling Publishing
% Canadian Manda Group, One Atlantic Avenue, Suite 105
Toronto, Ontario, Canada M6K 3E7
Distributed in Great Britain and Europe by Cassell PLC
Wellington House, 125 Strand, London WC2R 0BB, England
Distributed in Australia by Capricorn Link (Australia) Pty Ltd.
P.O. Box 6651, Baulkham Hills, Business Centre, NSW 2153, Australia
Manufactured in the United States of America
All rights reserved

Sterling ISBN 0-8069-4215-0

Contents

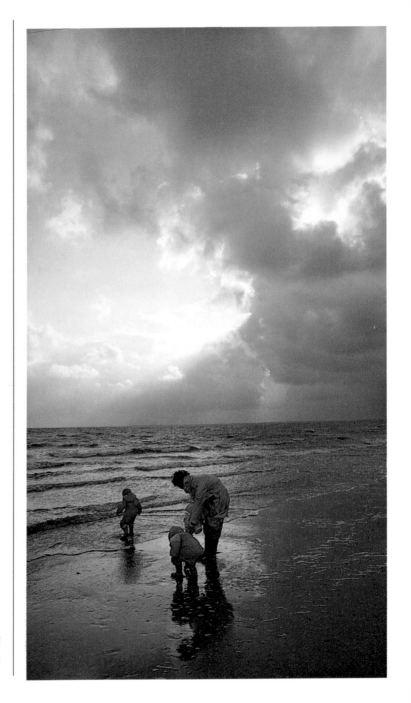

Our immune systems protect us from stresses and strains in our environment.

Preface

The environment confronts our bodies with many dangers. Bacteria, viruses, microbes, worms, and fungi threaten us from without; malfunctioning or dead cells from within.

All these foreign, sickly, or worn out organisms or cells must be removed from the body. That is what the immune system is for.

It is particularly important for us to know that we get sick when our immune system is not working properly in some specific way. The immune system protects us around the clock, so of course we should be willing to lend it a hand when it is under siege.

We have known for several years that our attitude can have a great influence on our immune system, in either a positive or negative sense. It is, within certain limits, up to us to manage our powers of resistance carefully. Everyone can learn to manage them. It is certainly important to know how to do this.

There are many methods by which we can enhance the effectiveness of our immune system: healthy living, eating a balanced diet, avoiding stress, being happy, engaging in sports, and making ourselves hardier. And if worse comes to worst—perhaps during flu season in the fall and winter—there are immune-stimulating medications we can take.

Unfortunately, we do not have a powerful control system to ensure the effectiveness of our strategies. The diseases from which we escape remain hidden from us. But take the common cold as a point of reference: you will find that you can reduce colds noticeably and that you can feel generally better, if you will just follow some of the strategies proposed here.

The immune system protects us from all the stresses, both external and internal, to which our bodies are exposed.

There is a wide range of ways to help your immune system in its work.

The Immune System

The Immune System: Our Body's Defensive Network

Every life form is protected from infectious agents by an immune system.

All life forms, whether flies, frogs, or human beings, have mechanisms to protect their health. The practical defensive strategies are most cleverly worked out at the higher levels of development of animal species. Humans, in the course of their evolutionary history, have developed an enormously complex, finely coordinated defensive system against various infectious agents. Immunobiologists throughout the entire world are investigating these wonders of nature.

The immune system is, to be sure, an organ in its own right—even though it is divided up among many locations in the body—but our constantly growing knowledge reveals that it in no way works independently. According to present knowledge, the immune system is instead bound into a network, together with nerves, hormones, and the brain, all in communication with one another. Our feelings and attitude are also directly involved.

We can help our bodies

The immune system consists of a complicated association of different organs, in which a permanent, lively communication takes place among the individual partners. We can learn to participate actively in these conversations, and so assist our immune defenses to accomplish their duties perfectly.

The Building Blocks

The organs of immune defense

It had been believed for many years that the immune system consisted of just a few specialized cells. Now we know that, on the contrary, it consists of many individual cells and organs joined together into a collective organ. Each component partner takes over different duties that are important to life; if even one component works imperfectly, a definite disease is expressed.

Our immune system is a complex association; individual organs contribute to its functioning.

The most important immune system organs

Our immune system is made ready to fight and perform its life-preserving duties at many sites:

- in the blood cells
- in the bone marrow
- in the thymus gland
- in the lymphatic system, including the lymph nodes, and in lymphatic tissue throughout the entire body.

The intestines and the skin also play a critical role in the defensive battle, because certain immune cells are located there that are in direct contact with the outside world.

The thymus is the "school" for the lymphocytes. In a

CARRIERS OF THE IMMUNE SYSTEM	white blood cells (lymphocytes) in the blood, mucous membranes of small intestine, and corium
PLACES OF PRODUCTION	in bone marrow and thymus gland
ANTIBODY MANUFACTURE	in lymphatic tissue in the intestines
DESTRUCTION	in the lymphatic system (lymph nodes, lymph)

child whose immune defenses must be built up for the first time, it is an extraordinarily important organ, but in the adult it atrophies.

The cells of immune defense

The white blood cells, the lymphocytes, play the role of the police in the bloodstream.

The first and most important function of the immune system is to recognize what is foreign and what is native: what belongs to the body and what does not. This function is assigned to certain white blood cells, the *lymphocytes*. Ten percent of all body cells are lymphocytes: in a grown man, their total mass is about a kilogram (2.2 pounds).

Distinguishing foreign from native cells is, in principle, not difficult for lymphocytes: every cell must be tested, through certain features of the cell membrane structure. After such testing by the lymphocytes, cells that are native to the body, and which are healthy and functional, are left to continue carrying out their functions.

Killer cells destroy whatever threatens the body

Dangerous cells will be marked, destroyed, and their structural information archived—so that the next attack can be easily fought off.

All cells whose presence and functionality cannot be satisfactorily accounted for will be destroyed by killer cells. Those white cells that have already engulfed a foreign cell, such as a bacterium, are also destroyed, since they have already fulfilled their purpose.

Those lymphocytes that organize and coordinate the work of the immune system are called *T-lymphocytes*.

If an invasion of foreign cells, such as measles viruses, has occurred, then so-called antibodies become necessary for combating them, a role for which the *B-lymphocytes* are specialized. With them, antibody production can be swiftly resumed, if five or ten years later the person is again threatened by measles virus, since some of these cells have been instructed to archive the structure for the appropriate antibodies. Appropriately, these are called *memory cells*.

If the lymphocytes have carried out their recognition test and are certain that they have a bacterium, a virus, or a cancer cell, they send out the alarm to raise the defensive troops by means of a messenger substance.

The most important among these troops are the *macrophages*, regular trash bins among the professional cell eaters. They remain in the bloodstream for only a few days, then settle in the liver, intestines, spleen, skin, and lymph nodes, and wait in ambush there where foreign particles must cross an organic "pass." As soon as they arrive, macrophages secrete chemical substances such as oxygen radicals, nitrogen-bearing metabolites, and lysozyme, with which they can cripple or kill bacteria and viruses. The phages (eating cells) that specialize in defending against bacteria are called *granulocytes*.

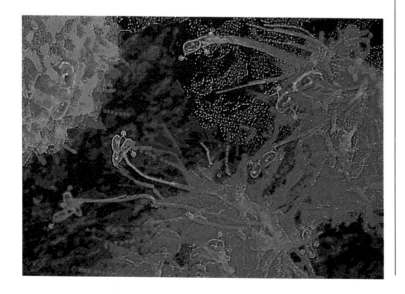

The phages (on the left of the picture, with "tentacles") are engulfing bacteria (the little rod-shaped structures on the tentacles of the phage cells).

The Cells of the Immune System and Their Roles

LYMPHOCYTES	Recognizing foreign bodies in the organism
T-LYMPHOCYTES	Organizing defense throughout the immune system
B-LYMPHOCYTES	Producing antibodies
MEMORY CELLS	Archiving the plans for making antibodies

Antibodies: our protective shield against infection.

Antibodies

The antibodies, also called immunoglobulin, are protein molecules dissolved in the blood. They are quite as important as cells in the battle against invading viruses and bacteria. They attach themselves to the enemy, such as a virus, by means of a specialized portion of their surfaces. If they are able to grasp the enemy, the eating cells will promptly kill it.

• The purpose of immunization is to stimulate the immune system in building antibodies that fight the sickness against which one is immunized. Through stimulation by special agents, the buildup of antibodies is encouraged.

We distinguish various types of antibodies: immunoglobulin G, A, M, D, and E. Each variety has different functions, and several of them play an important role in the strengthening of the immune system.

Immunoglobulin G—always there where it is needed

The most important immunoglobulin is type G. The majority of these antibodies patrol in the blood and travel from there to the aqueous humor, the spinal fluid, and the intraperitoneal fluid—sterile locations, within which disease vectors could become life-threatening.

The mother provides these antibodies to her unborn child. In the first ten to twelve weeks after birth, the newborn can carry on under the protective effects of the mother's antibodies—as long as his own bodily defenses have not yet been built up. After about the first three months, these antibodies are used up, while the first immunoglobulin G from the immune system of the child is still building up progressively.

Immunoglobulin G protects such sensitive places as the spinal fluid and the intraperitoneal fluid against disease vectors.

Immunoglobulin A—effective protection for the mucous membranes

Immunoglobulin A is responsible for the protection of the mucous membranes. If the mucous secretion is rich in antibodies, then the immunoglobulin is very strategically located, since most germs enter into the body by way of the nose, mouth, digestive tract, and mucous membranes.

Immunoglobulin A cannot pass through the placenta; therefore, the colostrum, the mother's first milk, is very important for the newborn. Immunoglobulin A contained in the colostrum is used by the newborn to protect himself or herself against bacteria and viruses.

Immunoglobulin M is a giant molecule, bigger than the others, that can reach the child in the uterus by way of the circulatory system. It reacts rapidly to any infection.

In normal situations, the immune system of the child starts up immediately after birth with the production of immunoglobulin M. After about nine months, the child has as much of it as an adult. It is neither possible nor necessary to lend assistance here.

Immunoglobulin D is less important in our present context. Immunoglobulin E very much the contrary: we assume that it has been primarily responsible for defense

Tip:
The nursing child is especially vulnerable to infection at the age of three to six months. Protect him especially at this time against avoidable dangers in the environment. This is also the correct time for his first immunizations.

In the first months of life, the immune system of the child is not yet fully developed. The child is dependent upon his mother's milk for many antibodies.

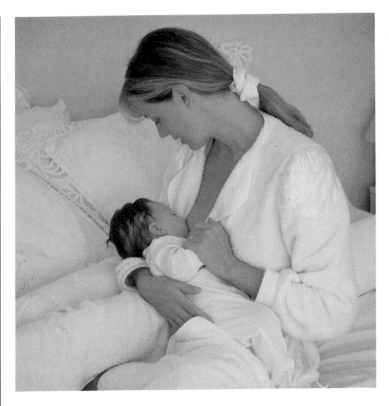

against worms. Immunoglobulin E has, however, another area of influence, one that is unpleasant to us, and often even life-threatening: allergy.

To breastfeed or not to breastfeed?

The effect of protective substances in mothers' milk weighs much more heavily than any possible harmful substances it might contain. For this reason, breastfeed your child, starting with its first meal after birth and for at least four months.* Then you can be sure that your child gets all the protection that you can provide.

*Recent guidelines in the U.S. suggest breastfeeding for at least a year is desirable. Check with your pediatrician for more information.

Communication Inside the Network

Despite all our research, the ways in which defense against diseases work are still not precisely understood. We know enough to say that there is a very complicated interplay between the immune, nervous, and hormonal systems.

The seats of government of the regulatory system are the brain (including the pituitary gland), the adrenal glands, and the immune cells themselves. A lively communication takes place among all these partners, in which not only the brain has its say: signals from the environment often stimulate the brain into action.

Hormones as bearers of information

Lymphocytes secrete hormones that are used as messenger substances, which, like all hormones, reach the brain through the circulation of the blood. In this way, immune cells in, for example, the big toe inform the brain of an infection of the toenail root.

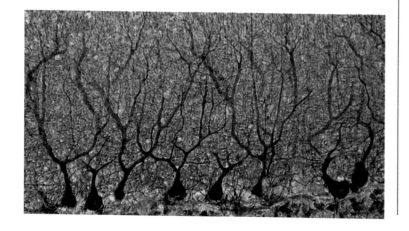

The individual organs of the immune system participate in a lively exchange of information. Over neural paths such as these, messages are passed on and commands are issued.

The stress cascade—a life-saving alarm

As soon as the brain becomes convinced of the seriousness of a call for help from the foot, it sends out hormones. If the problem persists, it sets in motion an entire chain of reactions that are called the *stress cascade*.

Everyone experiences stress. The sensitivity of individuals varies widely: one interprets the green light that signals him to drive down the street as a stress, while another would first become upset if he had just escaped by a hair's breadth from being run over. But in both the stress cascade has been set into motion.

The stress cascade is overall a helpful thing, frequently useful for saving lives. Stress is interpreted by the brain in terms of fight or flight. The order goes out to the adrenal gland: "Release cortisol!"

Stress mobilizes all the reserves of the body

Before we can bat an eyelash, a multitude of reactions are let loose in our bodies to make them ready for extreme life-saving actions:

> During stress our bodies remember back to a time when we lived like wild animals; this makes us ready for fight or flight.

What Happens During Stress

1. The heartbeat accelerates, which means that the pulse rate increases and blood is pumped more rapidly throughout the body.

2. The blood pressure is elevated.

3. The sugar content of the blood is increased to make extra energy available.

4. The skeletal musculature is perfused with energy-rich blood.

5. The digestive system and reproductive organs receive a diminished blood supply. They are not important in times of stress.

6. The blood supply to the immune system is considerably restricted. For this reason there is a heightened susceptibility to infection during stressful times.

The result is that the body is ready for extraordinary situations, especially where the skeletal musculature is concerned. The other side of the coin is that everything that can serve neither fight nor flight is turned down to just the "pilot light" during stress. Like the digestive and reproductive organs, the immune cells become inactive: no messenger substances, scarcely any activity of the killer cells and eating cells—and no antibody production. At this point the person is especially susceptible to illness.

After stress: Normalizing bodily functions

Normally, the emergency response fades away after a while; the man who escaped from being hit by the auto uses up his cortisol, his heart rate and blood pressure normalize, and his muscles are allocated less energy.

The regulatory feedback loop once again is stabilized at the accustomed level. The whole loop is a very finely tuned process that regulates itself. But like all regulatory cycles, the stress cascade is susceptible to disturbance and can be derailed.

The body's relaxation after a short time is just as necessary as the mobilization of the body under stress.

Disturbances of the stress cascade

Unfortunately, the regulation of the feedback loop often does not function as it should: cortisol remains in excess in the blood and leaves the body in a permanent state of excitation. This can be the case in:

- sleeplessness
- continuing stress
- depression
- anorexia

If too much cortisol is circulating in the blood, the body remains in a permanent state of stress—with fatal consequences.

The entire organism then runs at a higher speed—until it finds itself running on an "empty tank." Too much energy is consumed, without being used sensibly. Above all, the immune system becomes steadily weaker. When it can only operate in low gear, it is as if all the doors and windows were left open to bacteria, viruses, fungi, and cancer cells, which can then multiply unchecked.

Chronic stress causes illness. The body has no energy available to fight in its own defense.

Medications and the immune system

Medications also can suppress the immune system. Inasmuch as antibiotics and so forth are used in the treatment of acute illness, one must take this fact into consideration in determining whether it is better to use them or not.

Tip:

Many medications have an inhibitory effect on the immune system. Inform yourself about side effects, and discuss treatments— especially long-term ones— with your physician

The immune cells usually recover after the cessation of a course of medication. But each time, you should discuss with your physician whether and how you can further support your immune system during the course of treatment.

Medications and their effects on the immune system—what to watch out for

- Read information about the length of treatment on the medicine label and product information enclosure to see whether the medication has an effect on the immune system (for example, cortisone preparations).
- Discuss with your physician how long you must take a medicine, and whether a substitution of an immune-neutral medication (a medication that doesn't affect the immune system) is possible.
- Never take medications over a long time without a physician's instructions; even nonprescription remedies can damage the immune system, especially if they are taken in large doses (for example, aspirin).

How to Give the Immune System a Gentle Boost

Learn to reduce stress

Even if you feel truly healthy and fit, you may suddenly notice the onset of congestion, a sore throat, herpes eruptions, or shingles. The root of the problem could lie in an immune system overburdened by chronic stress, especially if you are a stressed out professional in a job that gives you no peace.

Stress has many causes

Personal events such as the death of a close relative, separation from your life partner, or pregnancy and birth of a child can also cause great stress on your immune system. Loss of employment, a new beginning in one's profession-

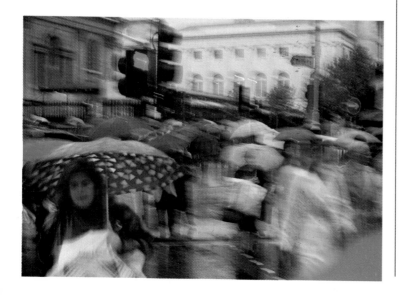

If life is hectic and a person is stressed, the immune system cannot work undisturbed.

Tip:
You must learn to deal with stress, since you otherwise will have to put up with unavoidable effects of stress on your health. For that reason there is no point in trying to avoid the effects of stress—you must learn to deal with them.

al life, annoyance at relatives, and being heavily in debt also can suppress the immune system.

Only an analysis of your individual stress factors can bring relief from the damaging effects of chronic stress. Become familiar with your own personal stresses. You can do it if you are entirely secure. Calmness is more useful for health than hectic running back and forth, or emotional ups and downs.

Meditation or another relaxation technique can help you if you find that you cannot gain control over your stress factors in any other way.

Sleep well

Sleep is not just a state that we fall into when we have nothing better to do. It has its own use and value, and people who lack it will after a time become sick.

Today, sleep researchers, physiologists, and biochemists can describe a host of processes that occur during sleep. Above all, they note how important sleep is for a healthy life and for enabling your body to have the power to resist infections.

The immune system brings improved sleep

A clear example of what happens during sleep concerns the messenger substances of the immune system, whose duty it is to transmit signals and orders among individual cells. One of these, interleukin-1, not only makes it possible for one to sink into sleep, but also serves as a messenger substance in the musculature and joints, to assemble the precise proteins needed to stimulate the musculature and various internal organs to work and the blood vessels to dilate. Overall, these processes lead to relaxation, recovery, and

In sleep our organs work undisturbed, important proteins are produced, and blood vessels are dilated. All this is important for our immune system.

the buildup of energy during sleep—all prerequisites for a functional bodily defense.

- Our immune systems thus need sleep urgently to accomplish their work.

Sleep and infection

When an infectious bacterial disease is contracted, more interleukin-1 will usually be released. You are aware of it: you immediately become tired.

When your temperature also rises at that time, the same cells that signal your need for sleep also release fever-reducing substances.

No peaceful sleep during stress

Stress hinders the immune system not only in the daytime, but also at night.

- The individual phases of sleep become shorter
- Sleep is not as deep
- The positive effects of sleep on the immune system don't occur.

If you work in the evenings, or sit in front of the TV and become excessively tired, you run the risk of being trapped in a spiral of stress-driven sleeplessness. Infections lie in wait for you. There is even a recognized syndrome that results from this sleeplessness-stress spiral: chronic fatigue syndrome, in which the individual feels tired all the time, which is accompanied by diminished capacity for work, emotional discord, various flulike symptoms, and chronic depression.

Protect your immune powers carefully, so that you do

Tip:
The as yet incompletely trained immune systems of children are especially needful of adequately long, undisturbed sleep. Be sure that your child does not see exciting movies or television just before bedtime.

Tip:
When you have an infection that makes you tired, you should, if possible, stay in bed. By doing so, you help your immune cells mop up bacteria and viruses.

not get caught in an illness-producing spiral of lack of sleep and stress.

Healthy laughter

According to folk wisdom, it is possible to laugh oneself well; at least, we know that it is healthier to laugh than to just mope around.

There is still no scientific proof that this is true. Nonetheless, we are now convinced that one's internal attitude can influence whether or not one gets sick—in acute infectious diseases that come and go, as well as in illnesses with an interval of several years between infection and the outbreak of illness, as occurs in AIDS.

"Laughter is the best medicine." According to the most recent understanding, this old saying should not be ignored.

Encourage the immune system

We might imagine that the immune system of an infected person with a positive attitude is in a position to hold the infectious agent in check longer. Ultimately, cheerfulness relieves and dissolves stress, and that strengthens anew the body's defensive powers.

While scientific research on cells and messenger chemicals is still attempting to find clear evidence for the claim, it makes sense that one should in any case cheer up the sick, especially sick children. Keep stress of every sort, even in the form of sad news, far from the patient, if this is in any way possible, so that the person may not be burdened on this account at that time.

Tip:
Keep sick relatives, especially sick children, in a good mood through encouraging gifts. Avoid passing on negative news to them.

Take up sports

One good way to encourage the immune system to work well is to undertake the kinds of sports that require the use of the entire musculature—endurance sports such as jogging, walking, swimming, cycling, and rowing. The aerobic sports provide your immune cells with more oxygen.

Various types of sports such as weight lifting or those requiring brief, intense peak loads such as bungee jumping are certainly rather harmful; like high-intensity sports, they place a burden on the immune system, so those would not be the choice to yield desirable effects.

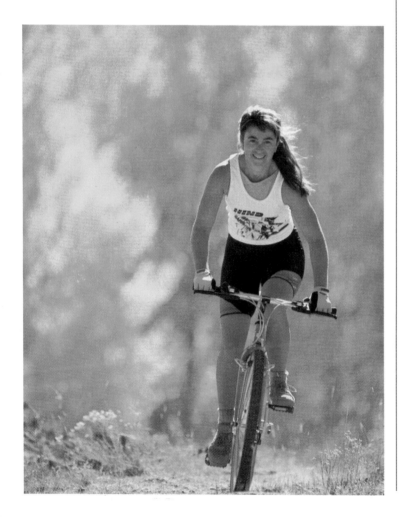

Endurance sports, which exercise the entire body symmetrically, provide your immune cells with more oxygen.

More oxygen through sports

Tip:
If you participate in sports, be sure that your body is uniformly exercised, that endurance rather than strength is developed, and that short-term peak loads are avoided.

The goal of gentle training is to improve the circulation. The better all organs are vascularized, the more oxygen they get. The increased oxygen supply throughout the entire body also reaches the immune cells. And the immune cells can fulfill their tasks better when they don't lack oxygen.

Toughen up in a natural manner

Hardening or toughening up (tempering) of the body against infection using water is an old, time-tested procedure. It has been shown that, as a result of the Kneipp cure, the amount of immunoglobulin M and of lymphocytes is raised; therefore, this method is valued as an addition to traditional medical-school style medicine.

An ancient means of strengthening the immune system: tempering with cold water.

As a result of this training to combat cold stress, more white blood cells and immunoglobulin are found in the blood. Scientists still do not know precisely how this process takes place in individuals. It is certain that the blood circulation is improved. Possibly the effect of water tempering is that the immune system learns to sound the alarm sooner. The earlier the immune cells are alerted, the

How to Correctly Make Yourself Hardier

- As a rule, use cold water on warm skin—for example, skin still warm from bed.
- Deprive your skin of heat for at most 30 seconds.
- After applying the water, the body must be warmed again, so go back into bed or bundle up warmly.

more easily they can conquer the intruders, before they have had an opportunity to multiply within the body.

For the hardening of a healthy person, but also for a person with a feverish infectious disease, the following complete washing can help:

- Wet a rough washcloth in cold water and wring it out.
- Smoothly and with constant pressure, while the person is standing, rub from the back of the right hand up over the outside of the arm to the shoulder, followed by the palm of the hand and up over the inside of the arm to the armpit.
- Continue on the right side of the back and buttocks and on the outside of the right leg as far as the back of the foot, and on the front of the body as high as the breast.
- Next, in a similar manner, rub the left side of the body with the washcloth, finishing with the soles of both feet. The head is omitted.

The Kneipp cure: a method of healthy washing

Tip:
If you can't do the complete washing, start with arm or leg washing and advance from there. If you are sensitive, weak, or old, you should begin with warm water, 95° to 102°F (35° to 39°C).

In a Kneipp cure, refined techniques can be learned—for example, treatments with cold, warm, or hot washings; partial or complete showers; baths or wrapping; and compresses.

The advantage of such a natural method is that the whole thing can be done without any medications or additional substances of any kind. This method places no burden on such organs as the liver and the kidneys.

Kneipp treatments are available in many health resorts and baths. But most of the showers and washings can be done at home. Kneipp cures can be carried out at home without difficulty, and entirely without side effects.

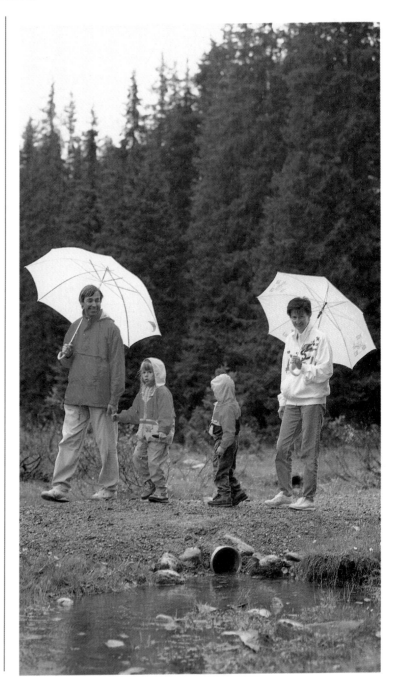

*By simple means, you can
help members of your
family strengthen
their immune systems.*

Active Health Protection for the Whole Family

Your Immune System's Strength Is Maintained with Vitamins and Trace Elements

It is very clear that we can best support our immune systems if we nourish ourselves as nature planned it for us omnivores to do: with a nutritionally balanced diet that is low in fat and rich in variety, one containing considerably more food from vegetable sources than from animal sources.

Unfortunately, our instincts today no longer motivate us to reach out for the proper immune-strengthening foods. We therefore have to consider the immune-weakening consequences of modern life when we plan for our family's health.

Many nutrients are not available in adequate quantities in our daily diet, and we have lessened their effectiveness through smoking tobacco or using alcohol. Other nutrients are now needed in higher amounts than previously was the case, because of environmental pollution. And finally, we have frequently replaced good nutrition with fast foods that have no nutritional value. We therefore must add knowledge to our instincts and ensure our immune system's protection with sound nutrition.

Environmental poisons and unhealthy eating habits hurt the immune system.

Vitamins

Good nutrition is the best support that we can provide for our immune system.

Vitamins have special significance for our nutrition, because they can protect us directly from bacterial and viral infections (perhaps through their protection of our skin and mucous membranes) or indirectly through their influence on the immune cells.

Protect yourself against cancer with vitamins

Vitamins serve in cancer protection and treatment. They play an important role in the repair of damaged cells, in some circumstances healing them before something more serious happens, before they perhaps develop into a tumor.

You may need to maintain a higher level of vigilance with regard to possible susceptibility to cancer if you are in one or more of the following situations:

That vitamins are important for our health has been known for a long time. Recently evidence has been found that they guard against the development of cancer.

- You are exposed to carcinogenic substances at work
- You are exposed to high levels of radiation (for example, through frequent air travel or proximity to radioactive materials) for job-related reasons
- You are a heavy smoker
- Members of your family who are related to you by blood have had or presently have cancer.

If you think that one or more of these situations applies to you, you should consult with your physician to see if you ought to be taking the antioxidant vitamins A, C, and E with selenium as medications. These would be taken for significant protection against several types of cancer.

Skin protection with vitamin A

Vitamin A protects the skin and mucous membranes. As long as the cells are well supplied with it, disease germs find no way in. However, if vitamin A is lacking, the membranes of the lysosomes (tiny organelles in the cells) burst, and the cells perish, leaving holes in the mucous membranes and skin. In the remaining wreckage of the cells, bacteria, viruses, and fungi can flourish, or the cells age prematurely and become susceptible to cancer.

A lack of vitamin A can have distinct consequences for your health.

The results of a vitamin A deficiency include:

- digestive disturbances
- coughing
- susceptibility to disease of the mucous membranes of the bladder and vagina
- dryness of the conjunctiva of the eye
- frequent head colds.

Vitamin A helps immune cells

Vitamin A and its plant precursor beta carotene are also necessary for the coordination of the immune cells with each other. Without such a vitamin, the immune cells weaken and remain lying inert in the refuse of half-dead bacteria and viruses, instead of cleaning them out.

To make the immune cells healthy with vitamin A is especially important if the immune system has been neglected or chronically weakened (for example, from taking certain medications; in young children; in diseases such as AIDS; and so on).

- Liver was once preferred as the source of the most concentrated vitamin A. But today you should avoid this meat because of its chemical contamination.

Tip:
Carotene, meaning vitamin A and its precursors, is especially richly supplied in butter, cheese, dandelion leaves, sorrel, carrots, apricots, spinach and lettuce, and in general in green and yellow vegetables.

The city-dweller usually gets an average of at most 1.5 milligrams (mg) of carotene per day, much too little under our present living conditions. From 15 to 25 mg of beta carotene per day would be optimal for protection against infections, heart and circulatory diseases, and for cancer protection. The daily dose for children is about half that of an adult's.

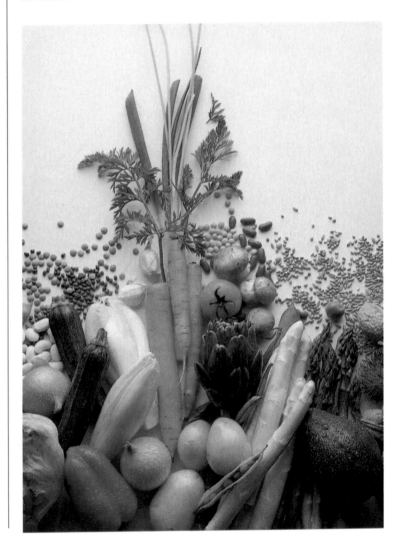

With fruit and vegetables you can supply your body with vitamins of many different types—and all without side effects.

To get 15 mg of beta carotene daily, you must eat:

4 oz (116 g) sorrel	14.3 oz (400 g) lettuce	9 oz (250 g) spinach
7.5 oz (215 g) carrots	21.5 oz (600 g) broccoli	6.5 lb (3000 g) tomatoes

The vitamin A supply from vegetables

Under some conditions, the vitamins you consume are not available for metabolizing, even though you have eaten vitamin-rich foods. That can happen if you have a very low-fat diet, liver injury, or a lack of bile. Estrogen preparations ("the Pill") and alcohol also diminish the availability of vitamin A. In this case you must simply eat vegetables more frequently. Doing so is not a problem, since there is no such thing as overdosing on beta carotene by consuming foods. That can happen only through long-term consumption of vitamin A tablets or capsules.

Tip:
Be careful to provide an adequate vitamin A supply, especially for children during a measles or chicken pox infection. They could easily develop a vitamin deficiency.

- Protect yourself and your family against bacterial and viral infections with green and yellow vegetables that have a high vitamin A content. Young children especially are helped by this in the autumn and winter. At the same time, you guard against cancer of the skin and mucous membranes for an extended period.

Vitamin E as a free-radical scavenger

Another vitamin that we have previously mentioned as a protective factor is vitamin E. Like vitamin A, E is an antioxidant, a scavenger of radicals produced by the splitting of molecules of water into hydrogen and oxygen, which are practically ubiquitous in our environment.

In our bodies, such products of splitting, called free radicals, play the role of destroying cells that have reached the end of their natural lifetimes. With air pollution becoming ever more prevalent in our environment, there are ever more of these radicals—too many! The skin, the eyes, and lung tissue must resist these overzealous pests that little by little attack cells that are not wholly healthy and functional.

When free radicals are dangerous...

Free radicals are especially dangerous to very delicate membranes, such as the cell membranes of red blood cells. Without vitamin E to serve as an "escort," the blood cells engaged in oxygen transport clump together and provide a basis for colonization by infectious organisms.

The opponents of free radicals, the antioxidants, are concerned with the repair of damage caused by the many radicals. If we have a vitamin E deficiency, cellular residues and fragments gradually accumulate. Visible signs of these casualties of radical attacks include the brown spots of pigment sometimes seen on the skin of older people ("liver spots").

...Vitamin E can help protect against cancer

Scientists suspect that unrestrained free radicals trigger cancer. Vitamin E can thus guard against the development of cancer, especially against stomach cancer. In the defense against infection, vitamin E, like vitamin A, is involved in the mobility of the white blood cells in their attack on bacteria. There is hardly any room for doubt that vitamin E is urgently needed.

Vitamin E is abundantly contained in cold-pressed food oils, margarine, whole-grain products, eggs, and nuts. During cooking, up to 50% of the vitamin E is lost, and light and oxygen reduce the E content even further.

Liver spots are completely harmless, and therefore are a purely cosmetic problem. But you can tell from their presence that the person who has them has a vitamin E deficiency.

Scientists now recommend 30 to 60 mg of vitamin E daily, much higher doses than previously. Many among them even advocate as much as 200 mg per day. 30 mg of vitamin E is contained in:

1 oz (25 g) corn oil	5.5 oz (150 g) hazelnuts
1.8 oz (50 g) sunflower seed oil	6.5 oz (187 g) margarine
3 oz (83 g) almonds	1.8 qt (30 liters) milk

Milk is not in the running as a source of vitamin E in comparison with vegetable fats and oils. It is practically impossible to get vitamin E in dangerous amounts from food.

Vitamin C protects cell membranes

Vitamin C and the trace element selenium work together with vitamin E to protect cell membranes. In contrast to vitamin E, vitamin C is soluble in water, so that neither can substitute for the other.

Vitamin C is concerned above all with the so-called basal membrane, the underlying network supporting all the layers of cells. When there is a vitamin C deficiency, this network starts to disintegrate, and in extreme cases it can become so thin that blood cells can slip through the interstices. That is the origin of the notorious disease scurvy, with which the sailors of earlier centuries, without fresh fruits and vegetables for months at a time, had to contend.

Vitamin C deficiency—at least in developed countries—is scarcely a danger anymore, but we need to consider a lack of vitamin C in regard to the immune system.

Vitamin C helps immune cells

Vitamin C is also necessary for the orderly functioning of

Tip:
If you think that your teenage or adult children are eating fast foods, give them almonds, hazelnuts, walnuts, and Brazil nuts more often. They can nibble their way away from borderline vitamin E and B$_6$ deficiencies, without your ever having to warn them about it.

Vitamin C deficiency: in the worst case, the consequences can be as severe as the notorious disease scurvy.

granulocytes in their attacks upon bacteria. The immune cells use up the vitamin C already present; during an infection, this leads within a few hours to a sudden decrease in vitamin C.

- For this reason, the speed with which the immune system can react to invading viruses, etc., is directly dependent upon the immediately available supply of vitamin C.

As a buffer for the vitamin C supply, we use the cortex of the adrenal gland, which is very well equipped: if cortisol is released during stress, it will at once be countered by the release of stored vitamin C. But be careful: under chronic stress, the storehouse can be empty.

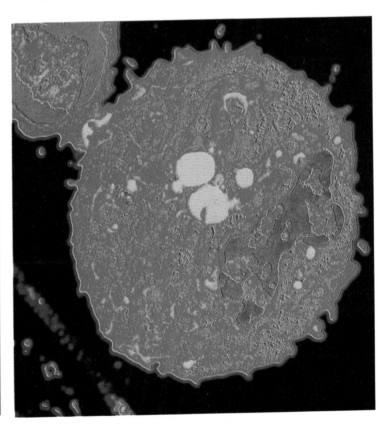

A cancer cell at 8000X magnification. According to the most recent knowledge, an adequate supply of vitamins can hinder the early development of cancer.

The daily requirement of vitamin C is currently estimated at 100 to 200 mg. Fresh plant products are almost the only reliable source of vitamin C.

100 mg of Vitamin C are contained in:

1.75 oz (49 g) red bell peppers	4.5 oz (125 g) lemons
2.1 oz (60 g) parsley	7.2 oz (200 g) oranges
3 oz (84 g) sorrel	10.5 oz (294 g) broccoli (cooked)
3.6 oz (100 g) green bell peppers	14.3 oz (400 g) spinach (cooked)
1.8 oz (50 g) black currants	2.2 lbs (1.1 kg) apples

Smokers need more!

Any smoker, drinker of coffee or alcohol, and any person whose body is severely stressed should include an additional 30 mg of vitamin C daily. Also, if you occasionally or frequently suffer from stomach troubles or gastritis, you must increase your vitamin C intake. Certain medications can also increase the need for vitamin C. Consult the labels on your medications to see if this is true.

- Since you cannot overdose on vitamin C, you can consume as much natural vitamin C as you want!

Vitamin C is sensitive to warming or cooking, and to light and air. Stored foods contain little vitamin C, as you can learn from the information labels on the packages.

For people concerned with nutrition, as for the gourmet, foods fresh from the market are unsurpassed! It's better to

Tip:
With a vitamin C intake of 400 milligrams per day, you can hope to ward off a beginning cold or the stress of a cold. In the following days, you can then slowly reduce the dosage.

Smokers and people who use coffee and alcohol need more vitamin C; their immune systems are weakened to start with.

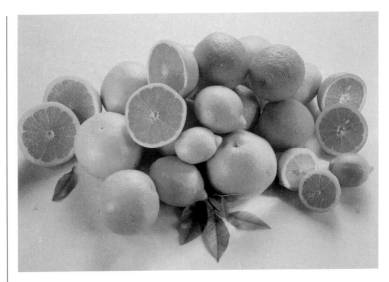

After fresh vegetables, fresh fruits are the most important source of vitamin C.

go to the store a little more often than to leave foods lying around in your refrigerator.

Vitamin B$_6$: Protector of the building blocks of proteins

Since there is no single place or function in our bodies that is without the building blocks of proteins, vitamin B$_6$ (pyridoxine) is essential almost everywhere—for the immune system as well. B$_6$ cannot be stored and is lost in the urine within a few hours of consumption. Anyone subject to high stress will frequently have a B$_6$ deficiency. Nervousness,

2 mg of pyridoxine are contained in:

5.2 oz (145 g) bran	9.8 oz (275 g) walnuts
7.8 oz (215 g) wheat germ	12.9 oz (360 g) hazelnuts
12.5 oz (350 g) soy meal	14.3 oz (400 g) bananas—about two
5.4 oz (150 g) yeast extract	bananas

irritability, and poor concentration are early warning signs that vitamin B_6 is in short supply in the protein metabolism of the brain and nerves. The daily requirement for B_6 is about 2 to 3 mg.

Trace Elements

Immune cells need zinc

Immunological disturbances often have their origin in a deficiency of iron, copper, zinc, or selenium. These so-called trace elements are indispensable for many of the functions of our bodies. Although more than 70 enzymes of the body require zinc for their functioning, at least half of the population is inadequately supplied with zinc. If zinc is lacking, the number of immune cells and antibodies in the body declines. As a consequence, the healing of injuries—for example, broken bones—is slowed.

We use trace elements for almost all of our bodily functions. Inadequate nourishment will lead to deficiencies.

Zinc deficiency—Who is at risk?

- young people who eat fast foods
- senior citizens who do not eat enough
- strict vegetarians
- pregnant or nursing women
- those with an illness-caused zinc deficiency (e.g., diabetics)
- women who take contraceptive pills
- athletes.

Zinc is present in muscle meats, fish, cheese, eggs, milk, and whole-grain products. The U. S. National Research Council recommends the following as the daily intake of zinc:

- for males age 11 years and up, 15 mg
- for females age 11 and up, 12 mg
- for women during pregnancy, 30 mg
- for nursing women, 15 mg

Although zinc is present in numerous foods, half of the population is inadequately supplied with it.

15 mg of zinc is contained in:	
3.2 oz (90) g bran	17.1 oz (480 g) almonds
12.5 oz (350 g) Brazil nuts	17.9 oz (500 g) walnuts
13.4 oz (375 g) Parmesan cheese	17.9 oz (500 g) whole wheat flour
13.4 oz (375 g) cheddar	17.9 oz (500 g) brie cheese

Tip:

Cheese cubes are better than potato chips as TV snacks. Instead of just having a bad attitude toward the empty calories of TV fare, make the snacks something that supports health and supplies the body with necessary zinc.

Concerns about enough selenium in the diet

With the proliferation of environmental poisons, an adequate intake of selenium becomes ever more important. Selenium deals with many toxic substances by reacting with them in the body to bind them into harmless complexes. Anyone who lives in an industrial region needs more selenium than a waitress at a country inn or a farmer. Precisely how much we need is still not precisely known; it is estimated that we need about 100 micrograms per day.

The daily requirement of selenium is contained in:	
3.6 to 7.2 oz (100 to 200 g) fish	about 1 quart (1 L) milk
3.6 to 7.2 oz (100 to 200 g) bread	3.6 to 7.2 oz (100 to 200 g) grains
a serving of meat	

Iron and copper

It has been known for a long time that we need iron and copper. Both are present in many foods:

Iron (recommended daily allowance 10 to 12 mg) is contained in: bran, wheat germ, parsley, soybeans, and eggs.

Copper (recommended daily allowance 2 to 3 mg) is contained in fresh yeast, bran, Brazil nuts, and eggs.

Garlic, the Immune-Strengthening Bulb

Garlic is one food that must be mentioned because of the comprehensiveness of its immune-strengthening properties. Its content of vitamin B_1 (thiamine) is very imprtant. We are somewhat undersupplied with B_1 under current nutritional conditions, yet with garlic alone, we can set to rest our concerns about this vitamin, so important to life.

In addition, infectious intestinal bacteria are inhibited by garlic, while the normal intestinal flora continue unharmed—in contrast to antibiotics, which kill the healthy intestinal flora.

Garlic has an unusually strong effect on dangerous protozoans (amoebic dysentery) and fungi, and on influenza and herpes viruses. Besides, garlic is effective as an antifermentation and antiseptic agent, and diminishes the uptake of harmful environmental poisons.

Tip:
There simply is no doubt that garlic is in many ways an especially healthy food. It has the greatest effect when you do not cook it, but use it raw. A large garlic bulb crushed in a garlic press and mixed into 9 oz (250 g) of cottage cheese is an immune-strengthening spread to put on bread.

Avoid Environmental Hazards

What skin and mucous membranes do

It is natural to desire smooth, beautiful skin. This is in accord with our instinctive understanding of its protective function. Healthy skin and mucous membranes do not permit passage of bacteria and viruses: the outer dead-skin layer and the sebaceous glands are involved as a mechanical barrier. For this reason we can afford to ingest so many bacteria: up to 1000 bacteria settle on each square centimeter of skin and there are up to a billion germs per milliliter of saliva in the mouth.

Few bacteria make us sick. Many varieties have evolved into a sort of "truce."

The skin is our foremost defense against attack by spores, viruses, and bacteria. If it is injured, danger threatens.

If a few disease organisms do trouble us, perhaps invading the respiratory system, they meet countless more sentries watching over our health.

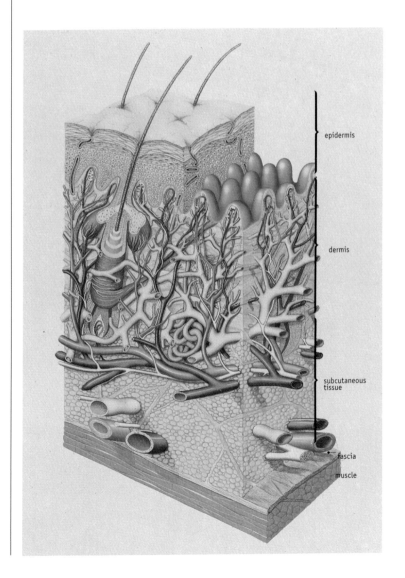

epidermis

dermis

subcutaneous
tissue

fascia

muscle

For healthy skin, bacteria pose no danger; a complicated cooperation between various defensive mechanisms takes care of that.

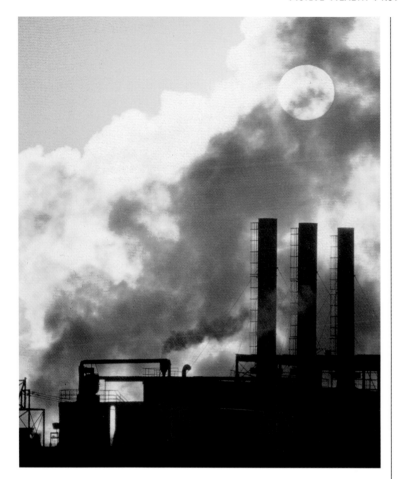

Industrial gas emissions and smoke from cigarettes damage the sensitive mucous membranes that intercept spores and bacteria that invade the body.

What intercepts invading germs?

- The tiny vibrating hairlike cilia, which transport the invading particles back to the outside
- The mucus, which engulfs bacteria and viruses
- The stomach acids, which render swallowed disease vectors harmless
- Disinfecting active components such as lysozymes, fatty acids, and lactic acid—for example in the nasal secretions, saliva, and tears

Every minute we are beset by hundreds of attacks of aggressive germs. All the above-named soldiers of the bodyguard normally watch over us without our even noticing. Compared to the number of attacks, it very seldom happens that a germ can find a loophole in the defense.

> The great majority of attacks by germs and bacteria are intercepted at the boundary of the mucous membranes, without our even noticing.

> The simplest defenses against bacteria and viruses are personal hygiene and care of the skin and mucous membranes, for people of both sexes and of every age.

Smoke

Among the most vicious enemies of the mucous membranes are the smoke from cigarettes, cigars, and pipes. In the present context we refer not to the long-term chemical effects, which can produce tumors after several years, but rather to the immediate effects.

- The cilia of the mucous membranes of the bronchi and the mucous membranes of the eye are also stressed, even by brief exposure to smoke.

Tip:
If there is smoking in the home, air it out as often as possible.

The smoker himself can reduce part of these damaging effects through increased intake of vitamins A, C, and E. The passive smoker also will be injured by smoke—scarcely less than the active smoker himself. The mucous membranes of children in particular can be damaged, and old smoke is no less irritating than fresh smoke.

Home climate

Try to maintain a healthy climate in your home: 68° to 72°F (20° to 22°C) is good. In rooms in which working and sleeping occur, the temperature may be a little lower.

During the heating season, the relative humidity of the air usually is too low indoors. If all the houseplants except the cacti wither, your mucous membranes will be damaged too. Cold viruses then have an easy time. A relative humidity of 40% to 60% is an ideal defense against them.

A departure from ideal conditions by itself hardly ever will make you sick; however, the skin and mucous membranes will be damaged. Then an invasion by a few cold viruses tips the scale.

- Your mucous membranes, like your houseplants, will find an air humidifier pleasant during the heating season.

UV exposure

In the stratosphere, the ozone is thinning out gradually—and in turn, ozone is increasing in the air we breathe. Both, for different reasons, are bad for our health and our immune systems. Ozone high up in the stratosphere has in general made life on Earth's surface possible: without the protective effect of this optical filter, UV (ultraviolet) radiation from the sun would impede all life processes on Earth.

The ozone layer in the stratosphere has already been considerably damaged. We all suffer from the resulting increased exposure to UV radiation.

Plant and animal life are highly sensitive to UV radiation

The chemical bonds that hold together proteins and the genetic materials of humans, animals, and plants are for the most part stable in the presence of visible light, which has wavelengths longer than about 380 nanometers. In shorter-wave light, especially in the ultraviolet-B wavelength range from 280 to 320 nanometers, these bonds break apart.

Under the bombardment of UV radiation, certain cells in

the skin, the melanocytes, are defenseless. Normally they protect our outer skin with dark pigments that we perceive as a suntan. Under UV irradiation, the genetic information in the melanocytes can be damaged, and the dark pigment may be deposited in an uncontrolled manner. Suddenly you no longer have protection; instead, the cells are mutated into that most dangerous of all cancers, melanoma.

- Because of increasing UV exposure, melanoma is on the increase among fair-skinned people and on the exposed parts of the skin of animals.

There is a growing suspicion that melanoma can develop especially readily in people who have been weakened by use of wide-spectrum antibiotics, sedatives, contraceptives, and tanning lotions, and by eating "empty calorie" prepared foods that are poor in vitamin B_6. Then even small amounts of exposure to UV light become dangerous.

UV light: Poison to the immune system

Damage from UV radiation extends from a weakening of the immune system to the initiation of skin cancer.

UV radiation damages enzymes that are essential for the normal metabolic activity of all cells and for all repair mechanisms. It is small wonder, then, that the immune organs are affected also.

UV damage is first noticeable in people whose immune systems are already severely strained, such as children and youth, pregnant women, the elderly, and anyone that has a disease. If you are besieged by diseases that are constantly troubling you—for example, herpes blisters—it is entirely possible that you have exposed your body to UV radiation.

- If you tend to get herpes blisters, you should avoid sunbathing.

- Cover your arms and legs and wear a hat or cap. Since we still know little of the dangers of UV exposure, we should avoid it at this point.
- It's possible that UV radiation may also have an influence on the progress of other diseases, such as AIDS.

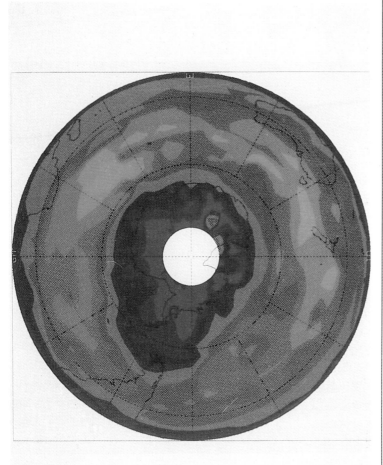

91–HC–783

Over the poles, as shown here in a satellite view of the Antarctic, the ozone layer is already so severely damaged that regular "ozone holes" have opened up.

43

Even artificial sunlight is dangerous!

Tip:
When your children are in the sun, slather them with UV-protecting suntan lotion! Damage due to sunburn is cumulative: damaged skin cells cannot recover in a lifetime!

Fundamentally, you should be cautious about exposure to the sun if you are susceptible to infections. The fairer your skin, the more dangerous the sun is to you—especially when the sun is high in the sky. Even modern so-called "safe" sunlamps give off radiation, and UV-A radiation is every bit as dangerous as UV-B. Suntanned skin may look good, but untanned skin lives longer.

- Do not under any circumstances be misled by false ideals of beauty and tan yourself under a high sun!

The damage of sun exposure accumulates throughout your entire life. The immune system can maintain the damaged cells safely under control for a while. But someday it will collapse under the cumulative load of all the little damages we receive from our modern environment. A weak immune system will collapse sooner than a strong one.

The tanning studio can be just as dangerous as the actual sun: all UV radiation causes damage to your skin!

You should, therefore, protect yourself from the intensive influence of the sun by means of sun protectants, by using sunblock in the mountains and at the beach. Be especially careful to apply sunblock to your children. Having many sunburns over the course of your life is apparently much more dangerous to your skin than exposure to the protectant chemicals. You should ask your physician about sunscreen preparations suitable to your needs: get ones that will help your skin, not the pharmaceutical industry.

Ideally, you should be able to avoid the sun's radiation by wearing suitable clothing and by staying in shady places.

Ozone in the air you breathe

The second danger from ozone is also a consequence of air pollution, like UV exposure itself. The burning of hydrocarbons, carbon monoxide and nitrogen oxides from automobile exhaust, domestic and industrial fuel combustion, and agricultural and garbage incinerators make and concentrate ozone where it isn't wanted—in the lower atmosphere, the air we breathe.

Ozone is used in microbiology as a powerful disinfectant: bacteria are readily destroyed by ozone. If air pollution continues to increase in the modern environment, people must take care that the same thing does not happen to them.

- Today, hardly anyone in the industrialized world can avoid the damaging and irritating effects of ozone in the lower atmosphere.

Ozone near the Earth's surface causes severe irritation of the mucous membranes. The damage to the cilia is irreparable.

Ozone is dangerous to mucous membranes

The first symptom of excessive ozone in the air is irritation of the mucous membranes of the eyes, throat, and bronchial tubes. Under the microscope, one can see that this irritation is accompanied by damage to the cilia. These organic injuries alone cause a reduction of immune system strength that should not be underestimated.

Important Data on Ozone

Natural upper limit:	60 to 80 micrograms per cubic meter
First physiological reaction:	90 to 120 micrograms per cubic meter
Ozone warning:	over 180 micrograms per cubic meter
Peak levels in Los Angeles:	as high as 1000 micrograms per cubic meter

The highest values of ozone concentration occur under the influence of sunlight and in periods of clear weather, and they are found, paradoxically, in regions with clean air, and not exclusively in urban settings.

People who suffer from respiratory diseases are especially at risk, and all those who breathe deeply outdoors: road and construction workers, athletes, and hyperactive children.

Long-term damage from ozone

The damaging effects of ozone, much like skin damage by UV light, are cumulative. Destroyed sites on our mucous membranes will not be repaired. Lost cilia in the respiratory tract cannot be replaced. The more often and the longer we are exposed to ozone, and the higher the ozone content rises, the more sensitive to infectious agents we will become.

- Leave your car at home as often as possible and travel by bus or bicycle.
- Make schoolchildren and their teachers aware that outdoor sports and games should not occur during the afternoon hours if ozone levels are high in your area.

The situation will improve only when everyone has understood this global phenomenon and laws protecting the environment are enacted. Therefore, it's important to try to influence your governmental representatives and make your health concerns known to them.

Tip:
During summer smog alerts, send your children to run around outside only in the mornings or evenings. During the afternoons, encourage quiet play indoors.

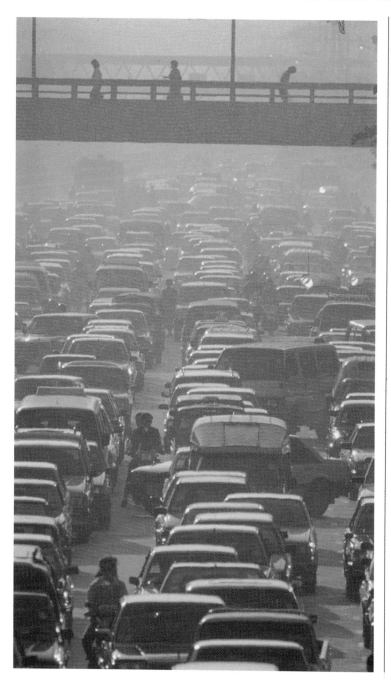

Heavy automobile traffic in the summer heat leads to a dangerous increase in ozone near the surface of the Earth. This effect is felt most of all a few miles away, in regions with clear skies.

Protect Yourself from Infections

When Skin and Mucous Membranes Become Permeable

When the skin or mucous membranes become permeable to bacteria, viruses, or spores, performance of the immune system alone determines whether or not infectious agents can be made harmless.

The immune system has several ways to deal with invaders that show promise of success. But bacteria and viruses have evolved a method of combating them. Unfortunately, there are even a few against which the immune system is utterly powerless.

The methods of attack of bacteria

Once bacteria have broken through the outermost defensive line, they give off enzymes that digest the membranes of the host cells. They use the contents of human cells as building blocks for their own metabolic processes. Many metabolic products of bacteria, the so-called bacterial toxins, affect our bodies as poisons. Cholera, lockjaw, and diphtheria are secondary infections caused by such toxins. The immune system is powerless against them; the assistance of physicians is required. Treatment is in the form of antibiotics and antitoxins, among others.

Unfortunately, the days are gone when bacteria could be combated by antibiotics without any side effects. Bacteria have learned to fight against antibiotics. This property,

Bacteria that enter into our bodies destroy cells. In the worst case, they then produce poisonous substances.

called resistance, can be passed on to the next generation of bacteria, and so on, to their distant descendants.

Since there are antibiotic-resistant strains of bacteria, it is often necessary to carry out a time-consuming search for an effective antibiotic, during which time the bacteria continue to spread in the patient.

Methods of attack of viruses

Viruses have no metabolism of their own. Everything they need for replication they take from the host cell, which eventually dies. It is important to the virus to find molecular groups in the host organism that it can pervert to its own needs. Only then can it attach itself. Thus a cold virus can attach itself only to cells of the nasal mucous membrane. The liver, for example, is spared from cold infections.

Once the virus becomes established, it takes command in the cell. It orders the construction of a host of new virus components; the young viruses then head off to attack new host cells.

Viruses take command in the cells they have invaded. These cells no longer work for our bodies, but for the virus instead.

Dangers from virus mutations

Viruses, like bacteria, are well equipped to fight against the immune system, especially against antibodies, since these are their principal opponents. Among the most troublesome of their battle tactics is the exchange of genetic materials, which contain information describing the constitution of the surface of the virus. Especially in influenza, in the true viral flu, and in colds we have to deal with the consequences of changes in the infectious cells' blueprints: immune cell antibodies do an excellent job, but the attachment points of the antibodies on the viral surfaces no longer fit! Thus the immune cells—and

The "cottage industry" of viruses is constantly inventing new variations of their genetic materials. The antibodies produced by the immune system are therefore mostly obsolete.

the drug companies—must quickly develop new antibodies or vaccines.

Methods of attack of fungi

The fighting techniques of fungi and the countermeasures of the immune system are not well understood. Fungal diseases occur mostly when the immune system is already weakened, when there is no functioning defense against fungal spores that are encountered.

At that time, the fungi that are already on hand on the mucous membranes, which normally would present no danger, multiply and are carried by the bloodstream to many different organs.

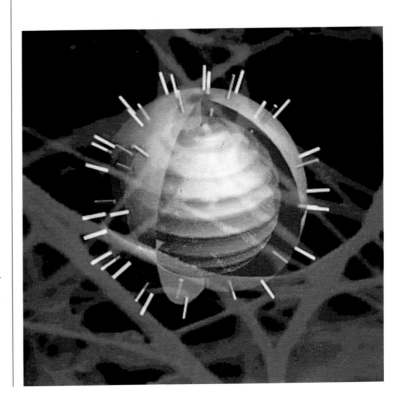

A flu virus has attached itself to a cell structure. If the cell fails to activate many antibodies, the virus takes command and forces the cell to work for it.

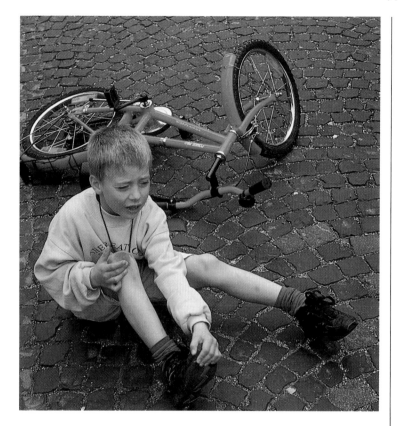

When the surface of the skin is broken and remains open, there is always danger that bacteria, fungi, or viruses can enter the body.

How the bacteria, viruses, and fungi invade

Bacteria, viruses, and fungi in principle all invade the body in the same way: either via the mucous membranes, through damaged skin, or, in unborn children, directly through the blood of the mother.

If the germs enter the blood via a puncture wound, bite, injection, or surgery, they completely evade the body's defenses: this way is therefore especially dangerous.

- The more readily viruses and bacteria get into the blood, the smaller the number needed for an infection!

• Disinfect any bite wounds especially carefully. Infectious agents there have especially easy entry into the bloodstream. Moreover, they can readily multiply among the dead and damaged cells of the wound. The same principle applies to abrasions and lacerations.

Distinguishing viral from bacterial infections

Viral infections are relatively easily recognized: they all develop according to the same game plan. On the other hand, bacterial infections are very diverse.

Almost all viral infections are similar at the outset. In bacterial infections, however, the symptoms depend on the kind of bacteria and can be very diverse.

Viral illnesses usually progress in two consecutive phases. The first is as a rule quite inconspicuous, and therefore not always recognized as the beginning of an infection:

1. A short period of decline, with muscle pains, headache, and joint aches, rising temperature, sometimes mild fever, and depression.
2. After a few hours or 2 to 3 days (in many diseases, even later), development of the virus-specific symptoms of the illness (for example, the spots of measles) and fever.

Usually viral diseases are associated with flulike symptoms.

Bacterial infections progress without much variation, but their symptoms are not uniform:

1. In most cases, the illness gets steadily worse from the beginning of symptoms to their peak.
2. Frequently the fever begins rather high.

Avoid infection!

An infected person is contagious. That is, he gives off infectious agents that are dangerous to others, and frequently does so long before his sickness has reached its high point.

The danger of contagion is therefore at a peak when the signs of illness are still barely noticeable: in a cold, before the nose starts to run; in AIDS, practically immediately after infection.

Viruses are present in the greatest numbers where they have just been liberated by the disintegration of host cells. Cold viruses live in the mucous membranes of the nose and mouth (and are sent out in droplets by sneezing and exhalation); intestinal viruses, in the stools; and the viruses of infectious liver diseases and of AIDS circulate in the blood. It is the same with bacteria.

Tip:
When a cold begins, stay at home and help break the chain of infection. If you cannot do that, then at least do not sneeze or cough on others. You are the only one who knows whether a cold is getting started inside you.

Fungal diseases—chronic and hard to diagnose

Fungal diseases of the internal organs are as a rule seldom acute, although over a prolonged time they can cause unclear symptoms of completely different sorts: tiredness, flatulence, and other chronic complaints. Such complaints can for a considerable length of time camouflage ailments that at first glance seem to have nothing to do with a fungus infection. Usually they are not diagnosed until all other possibilities have been eliminated.

- We can best guard against bacterial and viral illnesses if we take good care of our skin and mucous membranes.
- To guard against fungal infections, we must first of all support the immune system.

Fight with Your Own Strength

You can't observe the slaughter that rages in your body when bacteria and viruses invade—but you can feel it. Many of the participating immune cells pour out the very substances that tell the temperature control center in the brain: raise the temperature! This is very appropriate as a sort of liberation blow against infectious agents, since fever and fatigue leave us stumbling into bed—and rest helps the immune system in its work.

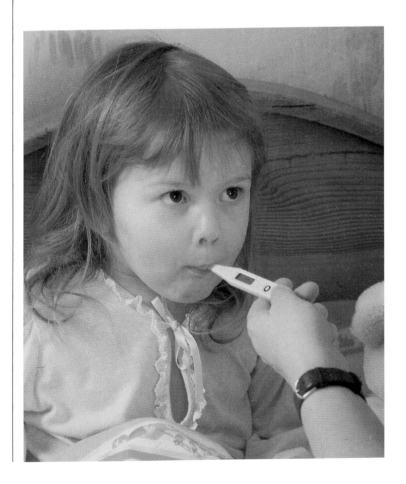

When a fever arises during an infection, it is proof that the immune system has been mobilized and the intruders are under attack.

Bed rest for infections

Bed rest is the first and simplest means of helping fight against most common infections, such as those of the respiratory system, the stomach, and the intestines. Don't deny yourself rest!

Drink a lot of fluids to help the kidneys in their work of detoxification. Extra fluids also can help in a flu infection by

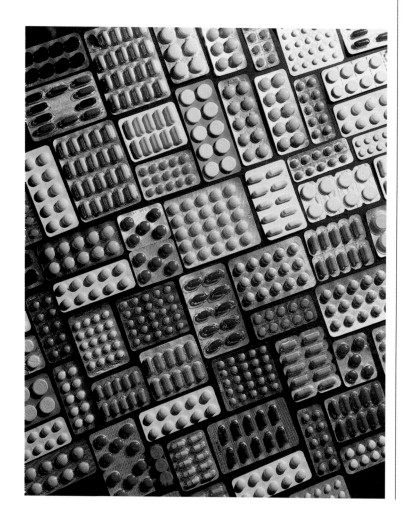

Medications are not very helpful during minor infections. Bed rest and lots of fluids are a sensible regimen.

thinning the mucus that can clog the nose and bronchial tubes.

Fever can help!

Don't try to lower all fevers by brute force. It is not the fever that is the problem—it's the disease. The fever shows that the immune cells are working; it also is effective in damaging the infectious agents, which are for the most part very sensitive to heat.

Fever naturally subsides

Of course, if the fever rises so high that it causes problems in its own right—such as too severe a burden on the circulatory system, vomiting, or fever cramps—it must be brought down.

This can be done carefully with leg compresses, which are quite as effective as medications, but without side effects.

This is how it's done: Wrap both legs from the knees to the heels with cold, damp cloths, and cover them with dry hand towels. Change the wrapping cloth when it warms up.

As a rule the temperature drops noticeably in less than a half-hour. If the temperature remains high or is alarmingly high, you should consult a physician.

Tip:
If the fever rises above 102°F (39°C), you should make cool leg compresses.

Antibiotics and the immune system

The immune system can be suppressed by antibiotics. This undesirable side effect can be countered by high doses of vitamin C.

Vitamin C is thus doubly important, since the vitamin C supply in the adrenal glands will be quickly exhausted at

Tip:
Consider carefully whether you should use antibiotics! In every case, supplement essential antibiotic therapy with lots of vitamin C.

the first bacterial stress alarm. You should therefore eat lots of fresh fruits and vegetables during a course of antibiotic therapy.

Since every antibiotic therapy brings with it the danger that more strains of bacteria may become resistant to them, one should take antibiotics only when it is truly essential. You could also develop allergies to an antibiotic that would make future use of it impossible, when it might be really needed to save your life! Also, you might become vulnerable to fungal infections as a result of taking antibiotics.

- For these reasons, you should not demand antibiotics. Do not pressure your doctor by telling him or her you have to get back to work.
- If your physician prescribes antibiotics immediately for every infection, ask him or her whether a harmless alternative might be available.

Only the immune system can help fight viruses

Viruses cannot be fought with antibiotics. Furthermore, there is still very little chemical therapy that is effective against viruses, and these medicines are not favored for use against the common cold because of their side effects.

Viruses within cells cannot be killed—at best, their multiplication can be stopped. The main work against a viral infection must be done by your immune system. The physician can only lend it a helping hand.

Nutritional changes to fight fungal infections

There are a few remedies for fungal infections that can have several side effects. If your fungal infection does not result from an immune system that has been severely damaged by illness, the best therapy is nutritional change.

Using antibiotics has the disadvantage of helping to create some bacteria lines that are resistant to antibiotics. Also, many patients become allergic to antibiotics and can't take them anymore.

Tip:
If you have a viral infection, use immune-strengthening strategies (sleep, stress reduction, and vitamins) and avoid everything that can place additional burdens on your immune system.

Protection through inoculation

People will not be able to imitate nature in all things for a long time, and they certainly cannot surpass it. But we learned long ago how to help the immune system fight against viruses and bacteria—through immunization (or inoculation). An inoculation or vaccination is a preventative defense against dangerous viral and bacterial infections. The defense is based on the immune system's developing antibodies when it comes into contact with bacteria and viruses—even if they appear in small numbers.

Because of this response, bacteria and viruses that invade later on do not make the immunized person sick, but instead are weakened or killed. Indeed, the best protection is achieved when the provoking organism lives and multiplies, since that means that the learning process of the immune system can be maintained for some time. But there are also germs that are so dangerous that they must be killed before they can be used in a vaccine, such as plague or cholera bacteria. Unfortunately, the immunizing effect is then smaller, so such inoculations must be renewed at intervals.

Inoculations and vaccinations protect reliably against a long list of dangerous illnesses.

Inoculation: Lifelong or short-term?

There are good, problem-free vaccinations against many viral diseases and against the effects of bacterial toxins—for example, lifelong protection against measles and long-term protection against yellow fever, poliomyelitis, mumps, German measles (rubella), diphtheria, and tetanus.

Inoculations frequently offer only short-term protection against bacteria such as typhus, plague, cholera, and whooping cough. There is no basis to the belief that bacteria and viruses are intrinsically controllable. They are unfortunately not, as we frequently learn to our sorrow.

Inoculations have only short-term effectiveness against many diseases transmitted by bacteria.

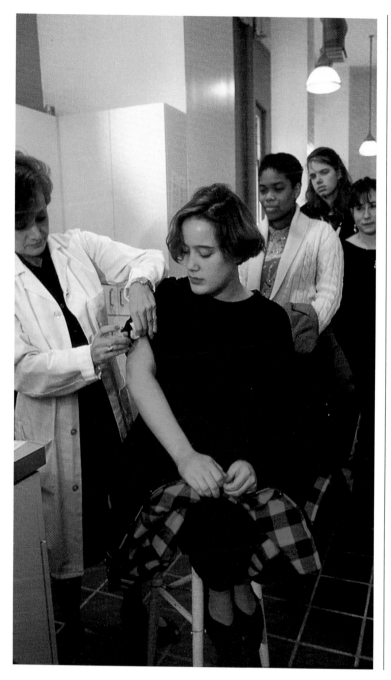

Inoculation is the safest known protection against infection. Since modern vaccines are benign, there is scarcely any reason not to participate in the recommended routine inoculations.

Inoculation calendar

Most countries have recommendations from the department of health or a similar body as to when and what should be administered. Most inoculations (vaccinations) are given during childhood. Check with your pediatrician and follow the timetable he/she recommends. The table below gives general guidelines used in the United States, but check with your pediatrician since guidelines change and the timing of some vaccinations can be varied.

Recommended Immunization Timetable

Hepatitis B	Three doses: At birth, 1–2 months old, and 6 months.* If the child hasn't received them in infancy, they may be begun any time in childhood
Diphtheria/tetanus/ pertussis (whooping cough)	Five doses: At age 2, 4, and 6 months, at 15 to 18 months, and at age 4 to 6 years. Tetanus and diphtheria toxoid boosters at age 10 to 12 years, and then every 10 years
Hemophilus influenzae type b	Four doses: At 2, 4, and 6 months.** Then at 12 to 15 months
Polio	Four doses: At 2 and 4 months, 12 to 18 months, and 4 to 6 years
Measles, mumps, rubella (German measles)	Two doses: At 12 to 15 months, then at 4 to 6 years or 11 to 12 years
Chicken pox	Two doses: At 12 to 18 months; & at 11 to 12 years

*Specifics vary based on the mother's immune status.
**Number of doses may vary, depending on the type of vaccine.

Problems Affecting the Immunization Calendar

ILLNESS OR PROBLEM	IMMUNIZATIONS POSSIBLE
Head injury/epilepsy	all; whooping cough carries some risk
Immune suppression	all except polio and tuberculosis
HIV infection	all except tuberculosis
Premature birth	all

Immunization under conditions of risk

In the past, many exceptions were made to the immunization schedule because of illnesses. Today this is in general no longer necessary, since the vaccines have become very compatible.

Beyond the routinely conducted immunizations, there are others that can sensibly be taken as needed; for example, during prolonged foreign travel.

Consult with your physician or clinic if you feel that you may be exposed to special risks.

As a general rule of thumb in the battle against infections:

Viral infections:
- Protect against viruses through immunization.
- Treatment of viral diseases is difficult.

Bacterial infections:
- Protect against bacteria by strengthening the immune system.
- Treatment of bacterial diseases is simple.

Since vaccines have become ever more trouble-free, there is scarcely any reason to avoid immunizations that could eventually save your life.

Immunization can protect against:

- Cholera (about 6 months' immune protection)
- Diphtheria
- Early-summer meningeal encephalitis
- Grippe, true viral flu, influenza
- Hepatitis A and B (liver inflammation)
- Meningococcal meningitis (inflammation of brain lining)
- Mumps, measles, rubella (German measles)
- Q fever
- Rabies
- Tuberculosis

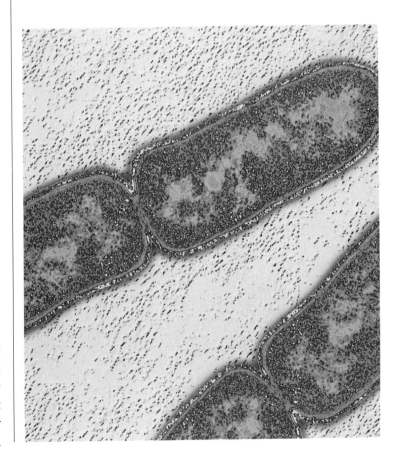

The tuberculosis bacterium viewed under the electron microscope. There are now effective vaccines against this and a long list of other severe illnesses...

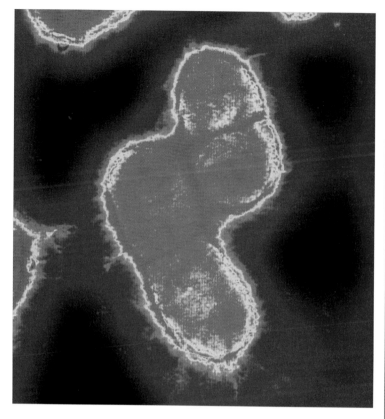

... but the list of illnesses for which we still do not know of any means of defense is distinctly longer: these include diarrheal diseases that are transmitted by coliform bacteria such as the one pictured here.

Immunization cannot protect against:

- AIDS
- Angina
- Relapsing fever caused by *Borrelia* bacteria (transmitted by ticks)
- Lyme disease (vaccine in development)
- Botulism (food poisoning by *Clostridium* species)
- Chronic fatigue syndrome (CFS)
- Creutzfeldt-Jakob disease
- Diarrheal diseases (except cholera)*
- Gonorrhea
- Flulike infections, parainfluenza, common cold

*A new vaccine against some deadly childhood forms of diarrhea (rotavirus) was approved by the US FDA in 1997.

- Herpes, shingles
- Caries (dental cavities)
- Legionnaire's disease
- Leptospirosis
- Listeriosis
- Bacterial stomach ulcers (vaccine in development)
- Necrotizing fasciitis
- Kidney failure from hantavirus fever
- Psittacosis (ornithosis, parrot fever)
- Yeast (fungus) infections
- Human erysipelas
- *Salmonella*
- Scarlet fever (vaccine in development)
- Septic shock
- Summer grippe
- Syphilis
- Soft chancroid (Ulcus molle)

Tip:
Protective immunizations must be brought up to date regularly, even for adults. Check to be sure your immunizations against polio (infantile paralysis) and tetanus (lockjaw) are still in effect. Renew your immunization against diphtheria.

It is plain to see that immunizations are the best defense against disease. They are highly effective and hardly ever stress the body.

There is a long list of standard immunizations that as many people as possible should get. The greater the number of people who have been immunized, the better the protection afforded everyone by immunizations—not just those who have been immunized. A large sea of vaccinated people protects islands of the unvaccinated in their midst. The danger that a local outbreak can occur becomes significant if such islands grow too large.

Tip:
Gently remind your friends and acquaintances of the importance of immunizations.

Build a buttress against infectious agents

Most of the infectious agents that cause serious illnesses can be outwitted. But you also should avoid the common infectious agents, since the sole benefit that accrues from their battle with the immune system is that you are able to escape from them. We should not succumb to the erroneous idea that the adult immune system becomes stronger as a result of conquering more infections.

- The best strategy against infections is to avoid them!

Everyday and occasional risks

Almost all infectious agents of humans arrive from outside the body. Therefore you should avoid, so far as possible, any environment in which infectious agents can be found, such as large crowds of people in the springtime during flu and cold season (risks: colds, influenza, flulike infections). Also avoid waters where swimming is prohibited (risks: diarrhea, lung inflammations, serious infections of the skin, and, in the tropics, worms or leeches carrying, among other things, HIV infection).

Also avoid dishes prepared with eggs, chicken, and questionable mayonnaise during hot weather (risk: *Salmonella* infection). Avoid undertaking travels in disease-infested areas (risks: cholera, malaria, diphtheria, encephalitis, and plague). Do not eat raw meats or drink untreated water in warm or tropical regions (risks: dysentery, typhus, and hepatitis).

Biting and stinging insects

In the United States, many species of mosquitoes, deer ticks, black flies, horse flies, and so on bite people, and many transmit diseases. In addition there are some dangerous species of insects and arachnids, including black widow spiders, scorpions, and killer bees.

We usually can escape from serious diseases by avoiding their infectious agents.

Tip:
Avoid the following: large crowds in the spring, polluted water, and travel in infected areas.

Ticks: The danger in the woods!

Tip:
Remove the whole tick within the first two hours after a bite! The Borrelia bacteria that cause Lyme disease first become dangerous after this interval. Try to remove the tick completely: a small injury is harmless compared to Lyme disease.

Ticks are dangerous, especially the deer tick (*Ixodes dammini*), which can transmit Lyme disease. Lyme disease can cause joint pain and stiffness, arthritis, malaise, chills and fever. Some patients develop neurologic abnormalities including

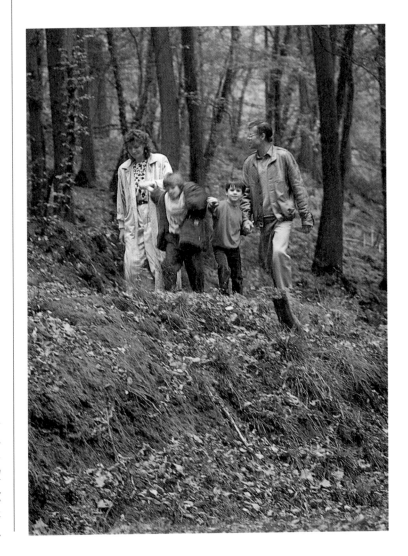

One can easily pick up a tick during a walk in the woods, especially in dense underbrush. Wear long pants and socks and check your clothing and legs carefully when you return from a walk.

meningitis and meningoencephalitis. Deer ticks are found in forested regions and even in backyards.

The disease was originally recognized near Lyme, Connecticut, but has appeared in over half the states in the USA, especially along the northeast coast, and in Wisconsin, California, and Oregon.

Ticks should always be removed promptly, but sometimes they are very tiny and hard to see. A raised red bump or whorl on the skin may be the first indication of tick bite. If you think you have been bitten, consult a physician and get tested for Lyme disease. Antibiotics promptly started will insure that the bad effects of the disease don't occur. A vaccine has been developed for Lyme disease also, and its creators are seeking FDA approval.

Danger from pigeon ticks

Relapsing fever can be carried by soft pigeon ticks (*Ornithodoros hermsi*) or body lice. The disease occurs pri-

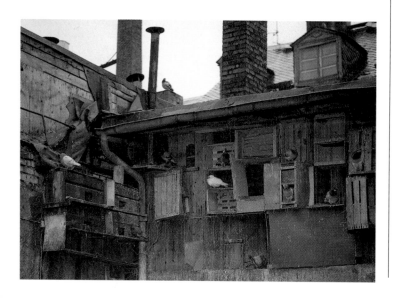

Pigeon ticks, carriers of tick-borne relapsing fever and allergies, lurk in ambush in dovecotes such as these.

Tip:
If your child should bring head lice home from kindergarten or school, treat him or her with a delousing shampoo according to the instructions, and check the other family members and playmates.

marily in the western U.S. The ticks come out at night and bite people. The ticks carry *Borrelia* bacteria that can cause fever, chills, headaches, and muscle and joint pain.

- Take care that the pigeon tick is removed. Laboratory diagnosis of a blood smear during a feverish period can diagnose tick-borne relapsing fever.
- Avoid the danger from biting insects by using insect repellants: lavender, laurel, and lemon oil repel insects for several hours.
- Nursing babies and young children can be protected by mosquito netting.

Infectious dusts

There are a few bacteria, viruses, and fungi that can be communicated through exposure to dust. You can avoid them, if you are aware of the places where danger may lurk.

Deer mice can carry hantavirus and are widely distributed in the U.S. Cotton rats also carry the virus. The hantavirus is mainly transmitted by dusty air contaminated with mouse or rat droppings, urine, or saliva. The disease produces flulike symptoms, high fever, difficulty breathing, kidney damage, and may result in death.

Tip:
Keep your children from playing adventure games in barns or sheds, where hantavirus may lurk.

Rodents can carry tularemia...

Tularemia (rabbit fever or deerfly fever), is a bacterial disease transmitted by flea bites from infected wild rodents or rabbits, or contact with infected meat. Tularemia can be treated with antibiotics. There also is a vaccine for people such as trappers or lab workers, who are at high risk because they work with animals.

...Domestic animals may carry Q fever

The danger of infection with Q fever is substantially greater. Sheep, goats, and cattle, cats, and wild animals can be infected with the bacterium *Coxiella burnetti*. The disease can be transmitted to people through dust that comes from the animals, ingesting contaminated food or milk, or contact with contaminated materials. Pneumonia and hepatitis may develop as a result, or more severe illnesses. Antimicrobials may be given to help control the organism.

Birds may carry parrot fever

Another form of lung inflammation can be contracted through contact with birds that are infected with psittacosis (also called ornithosis or parrot fever).

Especially if you have a weakened immune system, avoid the dust from tropical woods—for example, sawdust—and bird droppings, such as those of pigeons; otherwise, you could contract the fungal disease cryptococcosis.

The virus of the Newcastle disease of poultry can also cause an inflammation of the connective tissue in humans, or flulike symptoms.

A look at intensive medicine

Paradoxically, special dangers of infection await the person who must undergo an operation in the hospital. There are particular dangers inherent in intensive medicine; fortunately, they are not very common.

During recent years, contagious liver infections, yellow fever, and AIDS were accidentally transmitted through improperly purified blood and organ preparations. Some implant and surgical patients became infected with the dead-

Tip:
Do not under any circumstances breathe the dust from the cages of newly purchased caged birds!

Tip:
Avoid the vicinity of poultry farms if the newspaper has reported that an outbreak of Newcastle disease (fowl disease) is underway.

If you must undergo a scheduled operation, you can donate a supply of your own blood beforehand. This practice greatly reduces the chance of contamination with infectious agents from other people's blood.

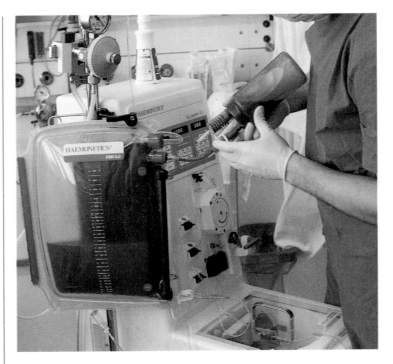

ly Creutzfeldt-Jakob disease. No one did anything illegal, but it was not avoidable either diagnostically or through sterilization.

Alarms have been raised by cases of AIDS infection resulting from transfusions. Blood banks try to monitor blood donations for problems. However, the possibilities of financial gain through blood and organ donation are so powerful that it is possible that from now on an uncontrollable gray zone will exist, within which an underground blood and organ "Mafia" will practice their deadly craft. There will never be 100% safety here.

In the long run, only a self-aware and critical attitude on the part of patients can encourage vigilance of the blood provider.

The risk of infection with the agent of the deadly Creutzfeldt-Jakob disease remains very problematical. At the moment, the infection itself cannot be traced in the blood donor or in the donated blood. That the risk is real is testified to by the fact that in November 1994 more than a thousand Japanese recipients of a specific lot of donated blood were affected when one of the donors died of the disease.

Precautions on trips

You can protect yourself by timely immunization against many diseases that may not be a concern in your own country, but are found in foreign countries. In some cases there are well-known procedures that protect you against diseases. Plan carefully and acquaint yourself with the possible health problems in the area you're going to before you leave home.

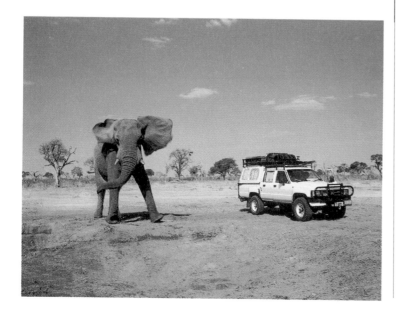

Careful preparation for travel—especially foreign travel—should include the planning of health protection.

Traveler's Guide to Infectious Diseases

Hepatitis A
Occurs in: Southern Europe, South America, Africa, Asia, and other warm places

Infection through: Contaminated foods

Precautions: Eat only cooked foods

Inoculation: Two basic immunizations; followup after ½ to 1 year

Diphtheria
Occurs in: Russia and adjacent lands

Infection through: Contact in crowds at airports and train stations

Endangers: People with weakened immune systems

Immunization: Before departure on the trip

Traveler's diarrhea
Occurs: Everywhere

Infection through: Dirty and insufficiently heated foods

Precautions: Taking the yeast Saccharomyces boulardii

Immunization: Not yet available

Hepatitis B
Occurs in: Southeast Asia, South America, central and south Africa

Infection through: Contact with infected blood

Immunization: Before departure

Typhus
Occurs in: South America, Southeast Asia, Africa, Hungary, Russia, Turkey

Immunization: Recommended. Protection lasts 3 to 5 years.

Yellow fever
Occurs: Sporadically in various countries; inquire before trip

Immunization: Required by many countries for travelers from yellow-fever areas

Plague
Occurs: Most recently, in India and Madagascar

Precautions: Bring an antibiotic

Tuberculosis
Occurs: Mostly in pockets of poverty and among the homeless

Precautions: Avoid direct exposure to coughing people

Cholera can appear anywhere that there is a lack of functioning water treatment and wastewater treatment facilities. If you have become infected during travel, you can in principle be cured readily wherever the appropriate medications are available. Be alert to particular outbreaks in the areas you're going to, and check to see if your polio or tetanus immunizations need boosters.

Cholera can appear anywhere in theory, but nowadays it is easily dealt with.

Be an Aware Consumer When Buying Food

No physician can evaluate what effect on our immune systems the totality of food additives, the metabolic by-products of animal medications, the various methods of food preservation, and disease vectors contained in foods might have. That they have an effect is without doubt! There is really only one sensible conclusion: Avoid processed foods, in which anything is possible!

Antibiotics

All animals raised for meat in mass-production "animal factories," including calves, pigs, turkeys, laying hens, chickens, and carp, receive antibiotics to protect them from infections, to increase their rate of weight gain, and to save money on feed.

Only part of these antibiotics is excreted; the rest remains in the meat, eggs, or milk. A waiting time is supposed to ensue before slaughter or before sale of milk and eggs, but it often happens that the animal or produce is brought to market as quickly as possible, in the interests of maximizing profits.

Such animal-feed antibiotics are apparently responsible

Antibiotic residues can nowadays be found in almost all kinds of meat.

for the increased resistance of many kinds of bacteria, for our allergies to certain antibiotics, and perhaps also for the increase in fungal diseases.

- Unfortunately it is fundamentally impossible to avoid antibiotic residues, but you can reduce the amount you get by limiting your consumption of meat.

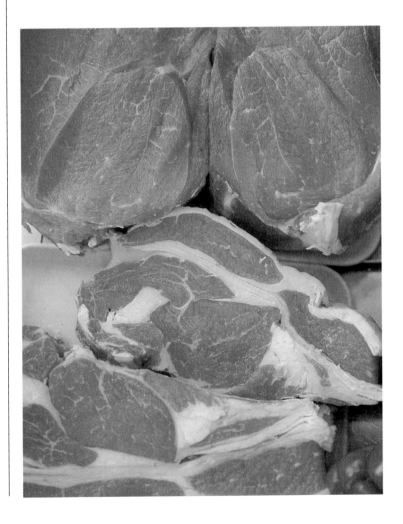

If you want to avoid animal medications, you must drastically reduce your meat consumption. You should at least beware of neck meat and hindquarters, where sedatives, hormones, beta-blockers, and the like are injected into the animal.

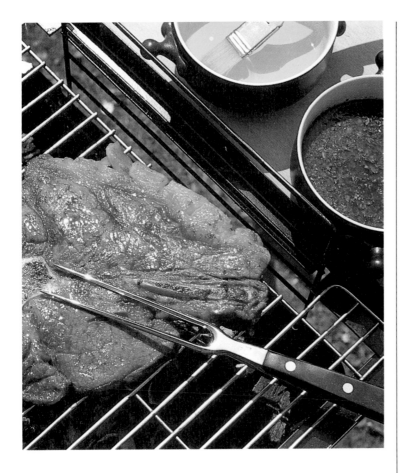

Barbecues can be a dangerous pleasure. The tasty dark crust can contain carcinogenic chemicals—especially if the meat has been preserved.

Irradiated food

Irradiation is used to kill harmful bacteria in some produce, such as tomatoes and meat. Irradiation is done using radioactive isotopes such as cobalt-60 or cesium-137. This process produces the cell poison hydrogen peroxide. In addition, it splits off highly reactive free radicals, whose effects in foods or in the human body are completely unknown.

It is likely that more irradiated foods will be on the market soon. Critical scientists fear that irradiation will be used to mainly make infected meat marketable, and are wary of the effects. The debate over irradiated meat is still in progress. Consumer groups want irradiated produce and meats to be labeled as such, so people can avoid them if they want to.

• Become an educated consumer and make your voice heard: exert your influence via letters to the editors of newspapers, state and federal elected officials, consumer organizations, and so on!

Preserved meats: Danger, nitrosamine!

Preservatives are another danger that is very bad for the immune system. Nitrites added to meat can be converted into carcinogenic nitrosamines. Such compounds are created very readily by the effects of heat, so be sure you don't barbecue any meats that contain nitrites..

Tip:
Never barbecue preserved meat or sausages! Heat, fats, and barbecue coals make preserved meats into a carcinogenic time bomb!

Infectious agents in foodstuffs

Salmonella bacteria multiply at an alarming rate! The victims of *Salmonella* infections are mostly the old and the very young, as well as those whose immune systems have been weakened.

Patients who have taken a course of antibiotics to fight other diseases are particularly at risk for *Salmonella* infection. Since the normal intestinal bacteria have been killed by the antibiotics and the digestive tract can barely produce the natural defensive substances, the *Salmonella* bacteria have a unique opportunity for explosive proliferation at such a time.

Salmonella—a hazard, particularly in summer

The disease carriers are mostly tainted chicken eggs that have been eaten or prepared raw, but they also can be chicken or pork meat. The food usually has been infected at the producer's. The bacteria reproduce prolifically up to the time of consumption, at a rate hardly delayed by refrigerator temperatures.

- Avoid raw eggs whenever possible! Beware of undercooked eggs, cook them well, and don't be deterred from doing so. Never buy eggs from a mass-production egg "factory."
- Ground meats should be eaten, or at least cooked thoroughly, on the day of purchase. Temperatures of 131°F (55°C) for an hour or more or 140°F (60°C) for over a half-hour, measured at the center of the cooking container, will completely kill all the *Salmonella* bacteria present.
- With prepared foods that you thaw in the microwave, you cannot generally be sure whether the *Salmonella* bacteria have been destroyed.
- Avoid contamination of foods and food preparation surfaces from the melt water from frozen chicken, and put the food preparation implements immediately into the dishwasher, or wash them with hot, soapy water.

Salmonella poisonings occur more frequently than one would think, and progress very painfully.

Tip:
Be on guard against Salmonella, especially during the warm season. Eggs, chicken, and ground meats can be especially dangerous.

Cheap meat: A time bomb

Over and over again, the media warn us about spoiled meat in the meat departments of supermarkets.

You cannot always see evidence of impurities in cheap meat. You should especially be aware that such meat may come from an animal that, during its short life, was stuffed full of hormones, antibiotics, vitamins, and other substances, so as to reach its slaughter weight in the shortest possible time. If you have decorated your plate with PSE (pale, soft, exuding) meat, be aware that all the artificial substances in it cannot have been inactive for very long.

Immune Stimulants and Immune Modulators

Fog, drizzle, and cold air—there are times when we wish for a stainless-steel immune system that isn't stopped by sneezing fellow humans or by an epidemic of flu. Any immune system can be conquered if it is under sufficient stress. On the other hand, scientists have found materials

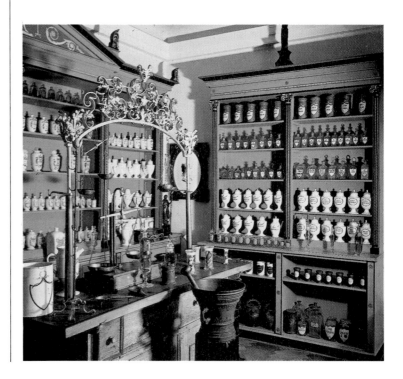

People have known about many herbal preparations and their effects on the immune system for centuries.

and methods of improving the performance of the immune system. Such substances are called immune stimulants or immune modulators. Many of them come from the plant world.

Herbal immune stimulants

The search for immune modulators has led to various plants that have been known to be useful in folk medicine for a long time, and has also led to understanding of what parts of the immune system they stimulate into operation.

Herbal immune stimulants strengthen our immune systems and help us overcome illness.

What Herbal Immune Stimulants Do	
Coneflower (Echinacea)	Multiplication of phage cells
Arnica	Multiplication of phage cells
Baptisia (wild indigo)	Multiplication of phage cells; better coordination of cells
Aloe	Multiplication of phage cells; better coordination of cells
Thuja (yew)	Better coordination of cells
Garlic	Improved assembly of enzymes used by the immune system
Mint oil	Improved antibody production in the mucous membranes after inhalation

Uses

Through herbal immune system stimulants, children, the elderly, and athletes can guard against infections.

It has been proven that immune modulators show their effects particularly when the immune system has been weakened or is at the limits of its protective ability because of stress.

- The elderly and children clearly will suffer less from colds and diarrhea if they begin taking immune stimulants in a timely manner before the cold season begins.
- High-performance athletes can keep a threatening infection at bay both before and during the competitive season, when the immune system is severely strained, by preventive use of immune system stimulants.
- Immune modulators, when taken early in a cold, shorten the illness and relieve its symptoms.
- Immune modulators shorten course of herpes blisters, relieve the itching, and help the eruptions to dry more quickly.

Many doctors have recommended immune modulators as sensible precautionary measures. Others deny every result. The immune modulaters have no side effects that you have to worry about.

Organ preparations

There is a long list of medications made from cow organs such as the thymus and placenta, among others, for stimulation of the immune system.

These are used in support of therapy during chronic infections, to improve the general state of health of the elderly, and as a supplemental therapy for cancer and rheumatic conditions.

Danger from BSE (mad cow disease)

Recently there has been much in the news about BSE (bovine spongiform encephalopathy, usually called mad cow disease). As of this writing, it seems likely that BSE is a transmissible disease that can cross species through eating of contaminated meat from infected cattle or other ruminants, contaminated blood products, etc.

Science has still not conclusively proven that the BSE organism is the cause of the new variant of Creutzfeldt-Jakob disease recently found in the UK in humans, but this seems likely. Creutzfeldt-Jakob disease is a serious neurological disease that affects the brains of those infected and causes muscle spasms, dementia, loss of higher brain function, and results in death.

The U.S. Center for Disease Control and similar agencies in other countries are monitoring the situation closely, as is the WHO (World Health Organization). The USDA (U.S. Department of Agriculture) monitors herds and has banned importation of cattle and cattle products from the UK.

Donor animals for organ preparations can be infected with bovine spongiform encephalopathy.

It is really not possible to say how high the risk of BSE is for people. But since the disease is a bad one, it is probably better to err on the side of being a little too careful.

- Beware of organ preparations from cows, particularly ones from the UK.
- Change to herbal preparations. As a rule, you will achieve adequate results.

Keep informed about developments by reading current information on BSE.

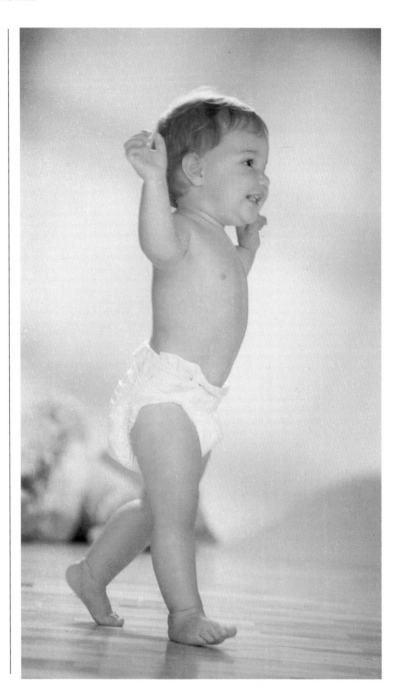

Children are especially susceptible to infections. Their immune systems must be stabilized.

The Weak Immune System

Natural differences in the immune response

Human immune systems differ from one another as much as all their other traits do. Just as one person is blond and another dark-haired, so they are also different in their susceptibility to infection or cancer cells. There are also differences that depend on sex and age.

Of course, the ease with which we respond to infectious agents can also be diminished by diseases, from the time of birth on. Often such immune defects are very complicated to diagnose and even harder to treat.

Immune systems are not all alike. Everyone has quite specific strengths and weaknesses.

The Immune Response in Children

Weakness of the immune system in young children is entirely normal and is a stage of human maturation. Building an immune defense usually begins at the moment of birth, when the child must begin to deal with invading germs on his own, whereas he previously could rely on protection by the immune system of the mother.

The most frequent infections of children are found in either the respiratory system or in the stomach and intestines: in the upper airways, as a head cold, inflammation of the mucous membranes of the nose and throat, bronchitis, and lung inflammations; and in the digestive tract as diarrhea, with or without vomiting.

Children do not yet have fully functional immune protection. For this reason, they frequently fall ill.

- Do not be upset if your young child frequently gets a cold. Instead, take comfort in the fact that his immune system is coping with the attacks of disease organisms and that it is learning how to do this with every hour that passes.

If you do not let your children play with other children because of the danger of infection, the immune training phase gets postponed into their school years. This is disadvantageous because of the time missed from school, and also because many illnesses can be more severe in older children. Confrontations with a wide variety of germs must take place in any case.

Infections are an important learning process

Tip:
Do not use disinfectants in your household: They are unnecessary or even harmful, since they inhibit harmless germs and thereby create opportunities for the dangerous ones to grow.

Your child's immune system uses its contact with the bacteria and viruses of our environment for its training. Not all of them cause diseases in the long run. Thus you should not attempt to shield your young child from common infections through isolation. Disinfectants may hinder more than they help.

- Of course, the diseases against which we must inoculate children are not the commonplace infections. You absolutely should take your child's inoculation calendar seriously!

The Immune Response of the Elderly

Flulike infections and influenza

The elderly must get used to the fact of their diminishing defensive power against infections, especially if they feel that they have been immune to the common cold or flulike infections for many years.

- You should resolve not to care for children who are sick with colds when the elderly are present, or else you must be very careful to protect the elderly. Elderly relatives should not be expected to care for sick children.
- The elderly can catch infections much more easily than they could have only a few years earlier; also, they do not recover from an illness nearly as quickly as children do.

Inoculations can protect against the true viral influenza, which has severe symptoms and can even lead to death. Since the virus constantly alters its form, it is necessary to get a new vaccination every year. Flu shots are recommended for the elderly, since they especially are at risk.

Food Poisoning

Contaminated foods pose a great danger to the elderly. The growing contamination of eggs and meat (especially poultry and ground meat) by *Salmonella* is especially dangerous to the elderly, since their immune systems can no longer deal with this sudden and threatening infection.

Take intestinal infections seriously!

Although a *Salmonella* infection lasts only one or two days, it is by no means free of dangers. Especially in the last few years, new infectious strains have developed that can cause a severe infection. The death rate from such infections has therefore grown accordingly. For this reason it is essential to report it at the first suspicion. A watery diarrhea and vomiting strike within 20 to 24 hours after ingesting *Salmonella*-contaminated food.

Tip:
If you are a senior citizen living in a home for the aged or group housing or you frequently use public transportation, be sure to get a flu shot every year.

Salmonella poisoning is no trivial disease. This is especially true when the disease is contracted by the elderly.

Previous exposure to the illness affords scarcely any protection against a new infection.

• Whenever you are under treatment with antibiotics you should avoid all foods that could contain *Salmonella*. Take seriously any intestinal infection accompanied by diarrhea and vomiting! Immediately visit or consult with your physician, who will probably prescribe antibiotics, which in this case is certainly advisable.

Hepatitis

The danger of contracting hepatitis (liver inflammation) increases with age. This is not, however, a consequence of heightened susceptibility, but of frequent operations. If you need an operation, you should consult with your family physician to see whether a precautionary inoculation against hepatitis A and B is advisable.

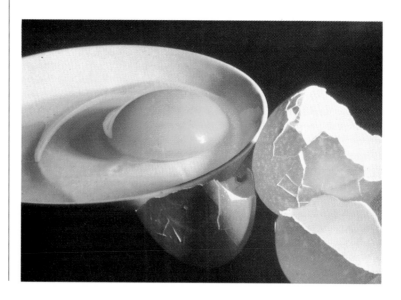

Eggs, especially those from "egg factories," frequently can be contaminated with Salmonella.

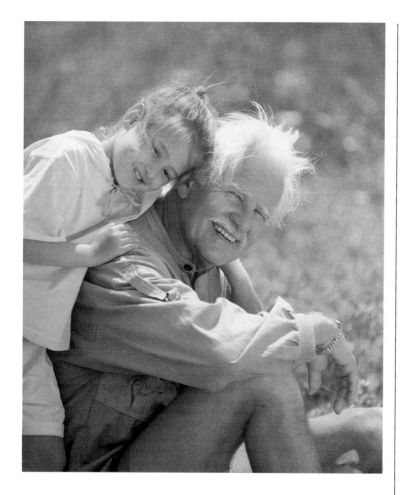

The strength of the immune system to fight off illnesses fades in later life. Because of this, the elderly can readily catch illnesses from children.

Tuberculosis

Tuberculosis is a true disease of old age, especially as a recurrence of an infection that took place in youth and has since then been in remission. Since antibodies to the bacteria are present, the symptoms are really not as severe as in a new infection. Frequently they are hidden behind other symptoms that older people might have for other reasons, such as coughing, breathing difficulties, and lack of appetite.

Differences between Women and Men

Women often have more stable immune systems than men do.

It has been found that there are differences between men and women in their defenses against infectious agents. Women possibly have more efficient immune systems than men, and this fact may be responsible for their greater life expectancies.

Men succumb to infections more frequently than women. Their susceptibility can most likely be accounted for by hormone production. Testosterone, which controls the development of the external sexual characteristics in men, can bind to lymphocytes. It can then hinder the lymphocytes in their functioning.

Purifying menstruation

It's possible that the cleansing effect of a woman's menstrual period causes a reduction in the infectious organisms in her body.

Estrogen in women discourages the production of antibodies, but is also evidenced in the heightened role of immunoglobulin in women. A modern theory of the immunological difference between men and women again raises the old idea of purification by monthly bleeding. According to this theory, menstruation is necessary and sensible as a means of eliminating infectious agents brought in with sperm.

- For these reasons it cannot be the goal of the physician to forcibly regularize irregular menstruations—they are evidence that a defensive battle against infection is already in progress. Here also, as with fever, the irregularity is not the disease, but a symptom or consequence of the disease. We must seek out the cause, not attack the symptoms.

Weakened Immune Function

Congenital and acquired immune weaknesses

Congenital weaknesses of the immune system are often severe afflictions that are beyond the scope of this guidebook. In the case of acquired immune weakness, precautions that support the immune system can only be helpful in conjunction with therapy. This principle also applies to damage to the immune system caused by x-rays and by treatment with immunosuppressants (medications that damage immune cells), as well as by viruses like AIDS and parasitic infections like malaria.

Continual stress through medications or x-rays can make the immune system collapse.

- In immune weaknesses resulting from medications or x-ray irradiation, there are many destroyed or weakened immune cells at the end of the treatment, but the immune cells can increase in number again. In that case, all immune-strengthening measures will speed healing.
- In diseases such as AIDS, we still do not know what assists or hinders the outbreak of symptoms. Care of the immune system may be the most important thing that the victim can do to lengthen the interval between infection and the outbreak of illness.

Tumor development

The connection between tumor growth and the immune system is still unclear. We know that both are dependent on each other, but we do not know the particulars. Certainly tumors get a chance to develop if the immune system is too weak to destroy the earliest onsets of the

It is not yet well understood how much a strong immune system can protect you against cancer. Modern medicine has mobilized all its resources to fight cancer.

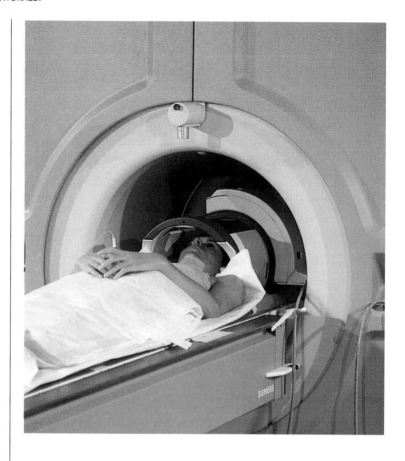

rogue cells. We also know that many tumors cannot be cleaned up by the immune cells, since they are not recognized as foreign to the body.

On the other hand, there are tumors that are induced by viruses, which give off the signal "foreign"; that means that the immune cells can seek them out to destroy them. On the whole, our knowledge of these matters is still very scanty. Precautions against cancer therefore cannot be targeted the way they are against flu right now.

When the immune system is damaged: Allergies and autoimmune diseases

The true job of our immune systems is to give us the ability to resist foreign intruders. Instead of this, it can sometimes happen that we become overly sensitive: one undesirable result is allergy.

Allergies...

In an allergy, antibodies are created to counter a causative agent, such as a virus. The next time one of these agents comes into contact with the body, the immune system reacts in an appropriate manner, according to what sort of agent it is and the route by which it enters the body.

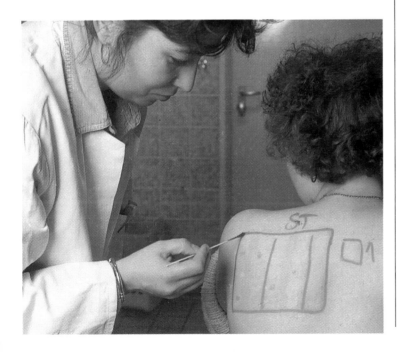

Nowadays, allergies are increasing alarmingly. Constant new stresses to which the body is subjected as a result of new chemical com pounds is the reason. The allergist or dermatologist seeks the identity of the irritating agent by means of skin tests such as these.

...Can have dramatic results...

Anaphylactic shock is the medical term used to describe the dramatic developments that can follow a wasp sting or an injection of penicillin, the consumption of protein, or treatment with immunoglobulin (for example, for snakebite). As a result of a powerful reaction of the immune system, pharmacologically active substances suddenly are released. They, in turn, lower the blood pressure, which can cause a collapse of the circulation. Take the following precautions:

- Carry your inoculation papers and information about your allergies with you, especially on vacation trips. In case of an accident, sting, or bite, a physician will have the information about which kinds of medications you must avoid.
- If you are allergic to egg whites, you should carry emergency allergy tablets with you. Before a meal in a restaurant or at a friend's house you should inform the others at the table of your allergy, and ask them to assist you or call a physician if it should become necessary.

Tip:
If you suffer from allergies, consult an allergist or dermatologist. In many cases she can free you from the troublesome symptoms through desensitization.

...Or long-term consequences

Less dramatic, but still important—in rare cases, even dangerous—is the slow release of the same substances as are released in asthma, nettle rash, and hay fever.

Substances that can trigger these allergic reactions include flower pollen, mold spores, dusts, animal hair, and certain foods. Your sensitivity to them will be noticeably heightened if your mucous membranes previously have been damaged—for example, by exposure to severe air pollution or smog, or by heavy smoking.

Autoimmune diseases

It can also happen that the immune cells make an error, with severe consequences. They think that they have found an enemy and hurl themselves at it until it is destroyed. But then it becomes clear that the cells that were attacked were native to the body. The physician calls this kind of attack an autoimmune disease. Diabetes, rheumatism, and certain forms of thyroid disorder are of this type.

The best known and most common of these autoimmune diseases is chronic polyarthritis. When one's own defensive system attacks the joints, the only help in many cases is a prosthesis. In addition, the thyroid gland (in Hashimoto's syndrome), the kidneys (Goodpasture syndrome), or the intestines (in ulcerative colitis and Crohn's disease) can be put in the line of fire by the body's defenses.

Science at a loss

There are various mechanisms that can lead to such reactions: genetic causes, or defects in the immune system, or similarities between bacterial attachment sites and the body's own cell structure. Diagnosis lies in the hands of the specialist; precautions are not possible.

No reliable method has yet been found by scientists to bring an out of control immune system back to order.

Of course there are medications that can hinder the immune system in its work—the so-called immune suppressants—but there is still no possibility of targeting their aim where they are needed. As a result, one can only suppress the entire immune system, thereby opening the floodgates to infectious agents. Even a slight cold may be life-threatening for patients who have been treated with such medications, since their bodies are no longer capable of fighting against even the most innocuous infections.

Autoimmune diseases pose a serious medical problem. Hardly anything is known about their causes and methods of treatment.

AIDS (acquired immunodeficiency syndrome) and multiple sclerosis

The classical methods and standard medications provide no remedy for autoimmune diseases. For this reason, the field of natural healing is once again being studied.

AIDS (acquired immunodeficiency syndrome) and multiple sclerosis are presently the best known immune system diseases. Just as with other related diseases that receive fewer headlines, they have not come under control using strategies such as those described in this book. But since it has been established that a strong immune system appears to delay the onset of sickness in HIV infections, we can hope that something will come from the areas of research of natural healing, which are beyond the standard medical methods of treating disease, that will be worthwhile in the battle against these life-threatening diseases.

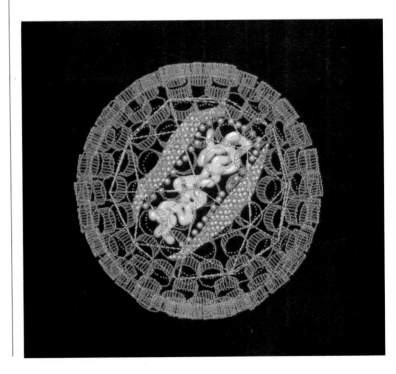

If the immune system is strong, the outbreak of the true AIDS disease can be delayed in some patients infected with the HIV virus.

Index

Photo Credits

Archiv für Kunst und Geschichte: 78.
Beiersdorf AG, 38. Oswald Baumeister, 51.
Das Fotoarchiv: 4, 90 (Thomas Mayer), 43 (NASA/DB), 66 (Henning Christoph), 70 (Eva Brandecker), 91 (Thomas Stephan).
IFA Phototeam: 1 (TPL), 24 (Fritz Schmidt), 59 (P.A.N.), 67 (Fischer), 87 (Heinz Koch).
Ulrich Kerth, cover, 28, 74, 75.
Mauritius, 34 (Rosenfeld).
Alfred Pasieka, 9, 13, 32, 50, 62, 63, 94.
Tony Stone: 1 (TPL), 12, 71 (Chris Harvey), 17 (Jon Bradley), 21 (Chris Noble), 39 (Paul Harrison), 47 (Ed Pritchard), 54 (Bob Thomas), 55 (Ralf Gerard), 32 (Lawrence Monneret), 86 (TSW).